Wonky

Margaret F. Oswell

Wonky
Published by Oswell Family
Cover Illustration by Susan Ballantyne
© Margaret F. Oswell 2015
Edited by Anna Cahill
Illustrated by Susan Ballantyne

National Library of Australia Cataloguing-in-Publication entry
Creator: Oswell, Margaret, author.
Title: Wonky / Margaret Oswell.
ISBN: 9780994288103 (paperback)
Subjects: Cerebral palsied--Australia--Biography.
 Cerebral palsied--Social conditions.
 Self-actualization (Psychology)
Dewey Number: 362.1968360092

All rights reserved. No part of this publication may be reproduced, stored in, or introduced into a retrieval system, or transmitted, in any form, or by any means (electronic, mechanical, photocopying, recording or otherwise) without the prior written permission of the publisher.

Wonky

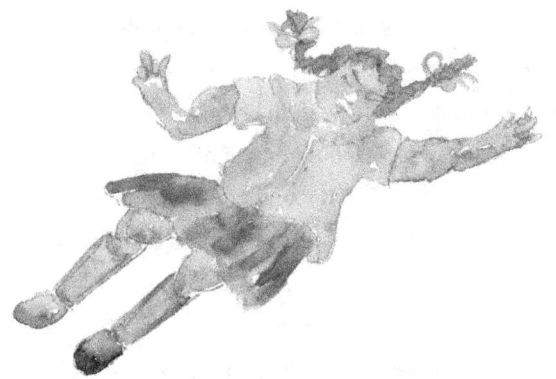

Reflections on the past

When is a smile not a smile?
When it is given just to show
How much you care
For all of us.
Although it was long ago,
I still remember Simon my brother standing there
Playing the violin at the funeral.
Showing no emotions although he was most upset.
I felt so proud of him.
Driving home I felt tired and sore
From hopping in and out of the car.
I told myself, with the rising of the sun
That I would be out of pain.
But the events of the day went so wrong.
I was greeted by someone with no compassion
In his heart.
He just stared at me.
Then he yelled "What's wrong with you?"
I made up my mind to
Venture back to your loving arms.
The place I love where
Most of my friends are.

Margaret F. Oswell, 2014

Author's note

All my life I've been called the 'wonky woman'. My mother called me that, my carers call me that. As I get older I get wonkier.

Wonky: not straight, crooked, askew.

Unsteady, shaky, feeble, wrong, groggy, tottering.

Wobbly, unstable, rocky, not functioning correctly.

Weird, whacked out, messed up, not working for no definable reason.

Overly studious, obsessed with details, nerdy.

So many random dictionary definitions, depending on whether you think it's old British slang or contemporary American speak.

Boy, I've got a lot to live up to! No wonder I'm even wonkier by the end of the week.

If you think about it, wonk is 'know' spelt backwards, or it could be an acronym for 'without normal knowledge. I know for sure that wonky is what I am, and wonky is what I shall be. That's pretty much what this story is about, how to grow up being a bit wonky and survive with a physical disability to have an independent life.

Disclaimer

This memoir is my personal recollection of how much of my life has unfolded, how I choose to perceive people, places, experiences and events. This is my truth. Others might view it differently.

"We do not see things as they are; we see things as we are"

– from *The Talmud*

Dedication:
To all those special people who have helped keep me moving all my life

Chapter One

I Come Into Being

I do not remember anything about my birth, of course, but my parents told me it was a 'breech birth'. That's when a baby comes out feet first. This was my very first mistake, the first of many in my life. The doctor was stuck in a traffic jam (no mobile phones in those days!) and the umbilical cord wrapped around my neck, depriving me of oxygen. As a result, my brain was injured to such an extent that, even when I was a few hours old, the doctors thought that I could be permanently disabled.

I was born at the Royal Brisbane Hospital in Queensland on 14 November 1956. At the time I decided to come along, my father was somewhere near St George, a large rural town six hours drive west of Brisbane in those days, along dangerous gravel and dirt roads. When my father heard there was a problem with my birth, he rushed back to support my mother.

After recovering from being told their only daughter would be permanently disabled, my parents named me Margaret Frances Oswell. This was a big name for me to grow into, but as time went by I knew that I could do so even with my disability. I do know that it never entered my parents' heads to put me in a children's home but I'm unsure if they went through a grief process like many parents with cerebral palsy infants do. Instead of celebrating the birth of a normal healthy baby, they brought home an infant needing extra special care.

I feel sure they always loved me but had no idea of the task ahead of them. Also, they were more hopeful about my ability to progress at a quicker rate than I did. One thing they both forgot, which has always surprised me, was that I had an emotional side that needed nurturing. They were always SO focused on improving me physically.

For some reason, I've never really liked the name Margaret, so mostly I go by the nickname 'Marg', except when signing important documents. This was just like Dad. At home, and to his friends, he was always known as Frank, but when it came to business affairs he was Francis. Being the only girl in the family, I was given Dad's first name as my middle name and I am quite proud of it!

To set the scene for my life let me tell you some more about my family. My father's name was Francis Bruce Oswell and he was born in Melbourne, Victoria on 11 January 1920. We affectionately called him FBO.

My mother's name was Glenda Mavis Oswell, nee Grundy (no relation to the Grundy of television fame as far as we know). Mum was born in Sydney on the 13th of September 1923. She was the middle daughter of Mr and Mrs Leonard Grundy. Mum suffered from high blood pressure as a child, a condition that caused her to faint often in the playground, and would impact on her in later life. As we grew up, we called her 'Glen' as well as Mum.

During the 1930s, Leonard Grundy and his family moved to Brisbane from Sydney. It was there Mum went to teachers training college, majoring in domestic science. After graduating, she was posted to a school in Kingaroy, an agricultural town north west of Brisbane. The poor thing told me that she hated living there, because of the social scale that existed. This town thought that young woman teachers were at the bottom of the social pecking order. She stayed in a boarding house run by two devout Christian women who frowned on single women.

It was at that time during the WW II that Dad met Mum. Dad was serving in the Air Force and living on the RAAF base at Kingaroy. On VE (Victory in Europe) Day he asked for her hand in marriage. She said 'YES' and they were married in the Ann Street Uniting Church in Brisbane on 25 April 1945.

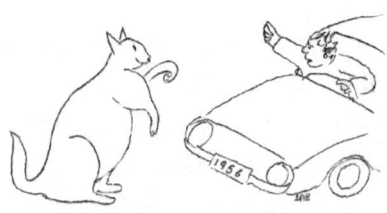

When he returned from the Second World War, Dad decided he did not want to go on working in the Commonwealth Bank. He studied architecture at the University of Queensland instead. His first job was to design large homesteads in the Queensland outback

- and I mean the REAL outback! During the early 1950s his job took him out to the bush every fortnight to inspect these homesteads.

The events of the first few days of my life told Dad that he would have to give up this roaming lifestyle, as much as he loved it. My mother needed him close to home, as I would need full time support for a considerable time. With my brothers and I to care for, my father decided to start his own architectural company. Dad's first place of business was in two small rooms, only a few metres away from where they were married.

Apart from my parents, I have two wonderful brothers whom I adore and love quite dearly. When I was born Simon was two and a half and Chris was one and a half. No, Mum didn't have two pregnancies in two years, they were both adopted, as she was advised against having a baby because of her hypertension.

Because of the constant attention I required, nanny Jeannette was also part of the family for the first couple of years. Her main job was to race around after my brothers, who were known to climb up on the roof many times before our parents wised up to their tricks. She often took me out in the afternoon sun while Mum had a quick nap.

We three kids faced some hair-raising situations over the years, but we always pulled together and worked our way through them, especially when one of us was in trouble. Really, our family numbered six because before my parents had children, they had a much-loved dog called Pam. She was a Wire Fox Terrier and an excellent friend to us all.

My father had a brother, John Livingston Oswell, who was two years older. He too went into the bank when he left school, remained working for them and made manager. John married Gwen Tweedale and they had three sons, Geoffrey, Michael and David. John and Gwen moved from Victoria to the Sunshine Coast, north of Brisbane, in 1975 after he retired. Sometimes on a Sunday we would go up to see them, occasions I really enjoyed.

Dad had a younger sister Dorothy who passed away at a very young age, maybe seven or eight. In all the years that I knew my father he never mentioned her name. It is quite remarkable to know someone for 46 years and you still don't know everything about them. This was the sort of thing that made me so cross with my father, the fact that when he found it hard to talk about something, he just would not speak about it.

He was a very clever person but we know now that he was a man who found it very hard to express his true feelings.

Mum's older sister's name was Beryl but everybody knew her as 'Peg'. She married a Brisbane man John Metcalfe and they had five children. There were two girls, Margaret and Christine who were a lot older than us. Ten years later came Donald, then Andrew and later Robert. Their ages were roughly the same as ours and, for the first decade of my life, they lived nearby. To a certain extent, I saw my girl cousins as two big sisters because I felt as if I could talk to them about being disabled. Sadly, they moved to Sydney in 1966 when John got a good job offer and we grew apart. Mum's younger sister Irene lived in Melbourne most of her life.

I remember Mum's parents quite well because they lived in Indooroopilly, the next suburb to us, so we would see them a lot. One of my earliest memories is of Grandpa Grundy walking down the main street of Indooroopilly making his way home from work. We all loved Grandpa and Grandma Grundy. They were very kind and happy for us to play noisily in their big backyard. When I was three years old, Grandpa Grundy retired from the plumbing business. Cataracts were growing over his eyes, so his sight wasn't too good. When they told Mum they had decided to leave the city and move down the coast she did not like that at all.

Fifty years ago, the 80 kilometre journey from Brisbane down to the Gold Coast was a long way. She was always concerned about them being so far away from her. Not only were they growing older but both of her parents had heart conditions and that really played on Mum's mind.

Knowing this, Dad decided to buy a beach house at Labrador, one of the northern Gold Coast suburbs, so that we could go down there most weekends to see how our dear grandparents were coping. When I was a small girl I always had a cold of some sort. Mum and Dad knew this house would also be good for me, so I could breathe some fresh sea air every week.

Living nearby Mum's parents meant it was far easier to get to know them than Dad's parents, who lived in Melbourne until I was nine years old. He told us stories about them though - like early in the 1900s Dad's father would pedal his bike every week from Hall's Gap across the Grampians (a striking series of sandstone mountain ranges) to Bellfield to visit Dad's mother before he married her. Dad's father was headmaster in schools around Victoria for a long time, unfortunately he brought the strict side of his nature home from school. He was a product of the era in which he grew up and was very proper.

One May night in 1965 John rang poor Dad to inform him that their very elderly parents would be arriving on the 11.30am plane from Melbourne the following day. Dad could not believe what he was hearing. When he and Mum recovered from the shock they asked us if they could have a few minutes alone. Obviously this was because they needed to talk about this problem and work it out.

When the plane door opened, and I saw Dad's parents for the very first time, I could not believe just how old they both looked. I don't know what my brothers thought, but it didn't seem promising to me.

By now Mum's parent's had moved to another house in Southport, so she suggested to Dad that they live in their old beach house at Labrador, which was now vacant, with a housekeeper, as they could not look after themselves. Dad stayed there with his elderly parents the first night and somehow managed to find them a live-in housekeeper the very next day. How was she so conveniently available? Well, it didn't take long to find out.

More often than not, things mysteriously went missing from my grandparents' house almost every week! One thing to go missing was a freezer. When Dad asked the housekeeper where it was she simply said it had gone up to Brisbane to get fixed and would be back before our next visit. And so it was. Dad caught her out again and again! For the next two years our lives were made so much richer by her antics and she really kept us on our toes.

The other thing I remember about this housekeeper was that she had a huge dog. It was an Alaskan malamute, originally bred for pulling sledges in the bitter Arctic winter. I thought that it was one of the most beautiful dogs I had ever seen! Standing right next to me she was nearly a metre high and weighed about 38 kilograms.

As we got to know Dad's parents we still found it hard to warm to them. Sadly they saw the world in a much more serious way than Mum's parents. They always talked about Queen Victoria and, whenever we went there, we were not allowed to make a noise.

Chapter Two

What Is Cerebral Palsy?

What is it that makes me what I am? Let me tell you a bit about cerebral palsy, how it affects one person very differently from another and the reasons for this. Cerebral palsy is character-building because you have to discover how much you can do for yourself and where you need support.

Back in the mid 1800s, English surgeon Dr William John Little was really puzzled by an undiagnosed physical disorder in newborn babies and very young children. He studied the condition and, in 1861, published the first ever paper on cerebral palsy, titled *On the Nature and Treatment of the Deformities of the Human Frame*. In this paper he described children having trouble crawling, walking, talking, or even grasping objects. Dr Little suggested this physical disease might be caused by a lack of oxygen at birth.

It surprises me that they did not start investigating sooner. I cannot help but wonder what happened to cerebral palsy sufferers before this time. Those who were very mild cases would have coped with family support, but moderate and severe cases would have been another story. I guess it needed a person of Dr Little's background to really notice the problem. As a child, he contracted mumps, measles and whooping cough, and later suffered polio in his lower limbs, which made him more aware of spastic disorders in children.

Dr Little's work was considered so influential at the time, that spastic cerebral palsy was first called 'Little's disease.'

Twenty-eight years later Canadian Sir William Oslar wrote the first book on the subject, called *The Cerebral Palsies of Children*. This book was a summary of all his lectures, presenting numerous case studies and possible causes of impairment. Not only was Sir William considered the 'Father of Modern Medicine' for his enlightened views, he is also credited as the very first doctor to coin the phrase 'cerebral palsy'.

This term, or CP for short, is used to describe a group of chronic conditions affecting muscle co-ordination and body movements. It is caused by damage to one or more areas of the brain while the foetus is developing, and can also happen before, during, or shortly after birth.

'Cerebral' refers to the brain and 'palsy' refers to disorders of posture and movement. This condition is not progressive nor is it contagious and, in the accepted sense, is not yet curable. However, combinations of therapy, medication and education now allow cerebral palsy sufferers to lead worthwhile and meaningful lives.

It was not until 1937 that recognition of cerebral palsy took its next major step forward, in the United States' city of Baltimore. Responding to a real need in the community, orthopaedic doctor Winthrop Phelps opened a children's rehabilitation institute for the treatment of youngsters with cerebral palsy. Today, this facility is known as the Kennedy Krieger Institute, in memory of President John F. Kennedy who enacted important legislation to care for disabled children, and an original board member and long time supporter, philanthropist Zanvyl Krieger.

In Queensland, there are about 7000 people with cerebral palsy. One baby in every five hundred has some degree of this condition. In other words a child with cerebral palsy is born every fifteen hours. These people do not have an intellectual disability, they can be very intelligent like myself, depending on the type of cerebral palsy they suffer. The vision of CPL, formerly known as Cerebral Palsy Queensland, is an inclusive world for all people. Across the state there are approximately 1800 staff and volunteers working with clients so that they can reach their full potential.

Where would I be without this wonderful association? Without physiotherapy I would not be able to sit. If I couldn't sit up I would never have seen the different things Mum and Dad were telling me about. And I'd have no way of going to school.

Basically, there are four types of cerebral palsy: spastic, athetoid, ataxic and mixed cerebral palsy. The type of cerebral palsy depends on the area of the brain that has been damaged. This, in turn, affects the muscle tone of the body.

Spastic cerebral palsy is the most common form affecting about 80 per cent of children and adults. This form is defined by tight muscle groups that cause quick and jerky movements. These people are often slow to move from one position to another and find it hard to hold and let go of objects.

I have athetoid cerebral palsy. It is caused by damage to the cerebellum, the processing section of the brain. This is the area responsible for ensuring that signals from the brain are smooth. Damage of this type can cause purposeless and involuntary movements, especially around the neck, arms, face and trunk. These movements make it very difficult to maintain body posture and nearly always interfere with speaking, grasping and reaching.

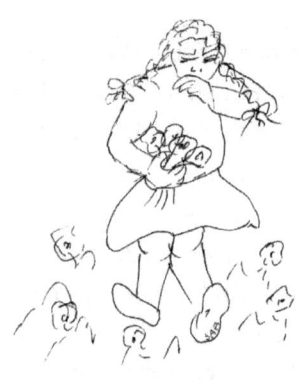

These random movements may also include tongue thrusting, which can lead to swallowing problems later in life. When I was a young child, my drooling was a real problem for my family. However, with speech therapy it became less so. Often, I would drop my towel while playing. When Mum and Dad saw me wiping the drool with my sleeve, they would yell "STOP WIPING YOUR MOUTH WITH YOUR SLEEVE, MARGARET". Yes, I was Margaret on these occasions not just 'Marg'!

Ataxic CP accounts for less than 10 per cent of those affected by cerebral palsy, causing poor coordination and depth perception. These people walk unsteadily, with their feet well apart and make a lot of shaky movements.

The fourth type, mixed cerebral palsy, affects about 10 per cent of sufferers. These unfortunate people have both the tight muscles of spastic cerebral palsy and the involuntary movements of athetoid cerebral palsy. Normally the signs of spastic cerebral palsy are seen first, and later the athetoid involuntary movements. In an average case, these uncontrolled movements increase between nine months and three years of age. This is the most common combination of symptoms but others also occur.

I had the double whammy of a breech birth as well as being born prematurely. When a baby comes out feet first, it has eight times the chance of having cerebral palsy. With the cord around my neck and the doctor stuck in traffic, the nurses simply didn't know what to do. Being premature, my lungs may not have developed fully, which also caused a lack of oxygen to the brain, and could have contributed to my condition. At birth, incidentally, I weighed about two kilograms, when the average birth weight was around 3.37 kg.

When the doctors at the hospital saw I would be severely disabled they decided to write little about me. Back in those days it was clear that these doctors and the general public believed that all cerebral palsy babies had mental retardation. The perception was we did not have a brain in our heads!

The doctors were so certain this was the case with me that they told my parents to put me in a children's home immediately and forget about me! They also told Dad and Mum that I would not amount to much. How rude and ignorant those doctors were to say such an awful thing. Perhaps they should have given me a chance to prove myself first. I'm please to say I have been challenging those wrong assumptions for most of my life.

One memorable example of this general ignorance occurred in 1975, when Dad was helping me off his 28ft yacht *Vert Gallant*. It was the Sunday before Easter, and he was preparing for the annual Brisbane to Gladstone Yacht Race. On the jetty a middle-aged woman had the complete hide to say to me "Don't be a chicken. You don't need to be helped off. Do it yourself!" I burst into tears after I got off, and Dad told her to shut up.

Thankfully, with my parent's strength of love and desire to nurture their very tiny daughter, they believed that the doctors were completely wrong. This love saved me from a terrible fate and allowed me to show people what I could achieve and do with my life.

Although the doctors were very negative about my prospects, they did record two things during my first year. At nine months, I could control my head and, at 12 months, I could tell Mum and Dad when it was time for a bath, using the little speech I had.

Chapter Three
Our Very Early Years

For the first 18 months of my life I didn't do much at all except eat whenever I was hungry, sleep a bit and play. Feeding me would take Mum hours every day as I was very slow to take milk from a glass eye dropper. Whenever Dad was home, he would help Mum look after me. His main job was to keep an eye on me every night while he did some of his own work. This was because I slept for less than 30 minutes at a time before being woken by a huge painful spasm that would make me cry my very tiny eyes out. A spasm is a sudden, involuntary contraction of a muscle. In other words, a muscle cramp. These contractions are usually harmless and stop after a few minutes, but are no less painful.

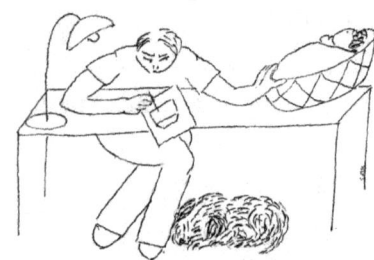

After he put my two young brothers to bed, Dad began the nightshift. He would send Mum to bed so she could get a few hours sleep before having to get up again about 1am. Then Dad had a few hours sleep. It took three years for my brain to start repairing itself so that I could relax enough to sleep throughout the night. Many of our near neighbours noticed a light on at all hours of the night at our house.

By the time I was nine months old, my parents were beginning to realise that the doctors at the Royal Brisbane Hospital were totally wrong. They noticed that I was pointing to different objects in my room and using my own special dialect with a sense of identification. At a year old, they were usually able to work out what I was trying to say, after a few attempts. On the first occasion, both Mum and Dad where just so overjoyed at this moment of discovery that they cheered with excitement.

When Dad told Simon and Chris that I was quite bright, they just walked away with their hands in their pockets like typical boys. I do hope that they were just as excited to meet me on their terms as I was to meet them. They could finally discover what I could do with my language and brain.

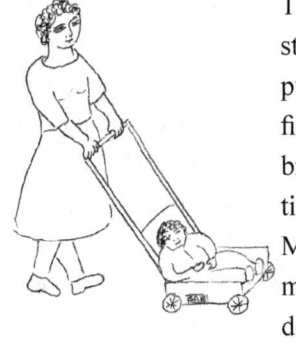

The next day Mum put me in my bright red stroller with brand new shiny wheels and pushed me out into our big backyard. For the first time ever she left me with my two big brothers. I was really excited but at the same time, I felt a bit scared because I didn't have Mum or my room to rely upon. My room was my special sanctuary where me and my rag dolls (I did not like other dolls, but adored rag dolls) would hang out together with our dog Pam.

I learnt how to enjoy myself with my brothers. Apart from being outside in the sun, which I still really enjoy, I very soon discovered that my brothers had decided not to show me any mercy. I thought to myself, *Well, I have my own language and if they want a fight I will give them one.* I suspect they were very surprised! All too soon Mum was back to see just how I was going and even she was astonished to discover just how much ability I had when competing and playing with my brothers.

While playing on the grass, I practiced my crawling more and more. One day I made my own way down the stroller ramp and out into the backyard. Now, my parents had suspected I was up to something during my backyard time but they didn't know what. On this occasion both parents and our nanny Jeanette were looking everywhere for me for 15 minutes. When Mum did find me, boy my brothers and I knew about it.

My two brothers are physically and emotionally completely different to each other. I guess this is because they are adopted. Mum and Dad gave them a stable loving home life while caring for me until I could do things for myself. For this I am eternally grateful. Getting to know Simon and Chris was a pleasure. I am very pleased that I can call them my brothers, will always be pleased to do so. After six decades as brothers and sister we have seen life at its best and life at its worst.

Simon James Oswell, was born on 15 March 1954 and he must have come from a musical family, as it appears that he was born with a musical instrument in hand. From the earliest day I can remember he was always humming to himself.

He was the brightest of the three of us. For example, he quickly learned to follow the ways of Frank and Glen. One Saturday afternoon we were visiting Mum's parents and he decided to pull their lawnmower apart, with Chris watching and Pam running around barking. When our parents saw what he was doing Dad went down and gave him quite a hiding. All Grandpa could do was laugh and tell Dad and Mum he would be only too pleased to fix the mower up. After that we all agreed that Simon was curious, a tinkerer and adventurer, and therefore 'a real Oswell'!

Christopher John Oswell was born on 16 April 1955, just 13 months younger than Simon. I sometimes wonder if my arrival into this world, and the degree of attention that my cerebral palsy demanded, had an effect on Chris as the middle child because he was only a year old at that time. He was a very physical little boy, very attracted to outdoor exploration, whether it be under a rock or up a tree, and making mud pies was always his specialty. He and I delighted in this fun, and Simon would join in too.

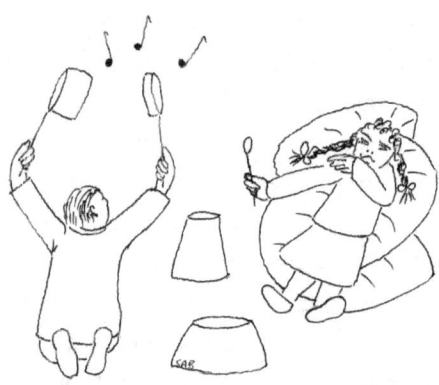

Chris preferred hands-on learning to the more serious side of education and will always be like that. When he was two, Chris used to bang household items together, which made me laugh uncontrollably. We didn't have Simon's musical ability and it might not have been pleasing to the ear, but at least we were good at it! With my help he turned into a real Oswell as well.

During my very early years the people outside our family that I most remember were the neighbours to our left. Their house was a double-story weatherboard place in a state of neglect and always looked as if it were falling down. Mrs Stitt, or Stitty as we used to call her, was a great friend of ours. The youngest of her eight kids was born the same day as me, so I felt quite close to her. She and a few of her young brothers and sisters would come over sometimes and play with us.

By this time Simon and Chris could sort of understand my weird and wonderful dialect. This meant I could tell them when I wanted my stroller pushed forward or backwards, and when I wanted to play or perhaps hit one of the other children. Just like all kids, we were growing up fast and each of us started doing more and more things according to our ages.

When I was about 18 months of age, Dad and Mum noticed that there was a need for some other support in my life. This took them on a journey to find a training centre for children with cerebral palsy. Much to my parents' relief they found the Queensland Spastic Welfare League in New Farm, an inner city suburb 45 minutes drive from our place.

Mum rang the medical superintendent to make enquiries about my long-term care and training. This really opened up my whole life.

I don't remember anything about going to New Farm for the very first time. I imagine that I was quite frightened because before this, I had just been at home with my family, neighbours and one or two other family friends. Now here I was, my parents talking to foreign people in an unfamiliar place who were going to assess my disability to see what services and support these strangers could provide to help me live my life.

I spent an hour with the doctor to determine what type of cerebral palsy I had and what my needs were. Then began a tense six week wait for my parents to see if I had been accepted as a long-term client. The good news was that Mum got the go-ahead to take me to New Farm every month for physiotherapy and, at the same time, learn how to work with me at home. She, in turn, was able to show Dad, who spent a great deal of time helping me with the exercises.

The relatively new organisation that had accepted me in the late 1950s has undergone many changes, including its name. On the 50th anniversary of the league, the name was changed because most people felt the word 'spastic' was distasteful. So, on 16 March 1998, the organisation became the Queensland Cerebral Palsy Welfare League. At that time I did not have an opinion. Thinking about this subject a bit more, I too think it is a more suitable name because the word 'spastic' only embraces one group of cerebral palsy people instead of the whole Queensland cerebral palsy population.

The league often uses a dragonfly as a symbol of cerebral palsy to raise understanding in the wider community. I really like this analogy. There are over 320 different kinds of dragonflies in Australia alone (more than 4500 in the world), yet even with a broken wing or a missing leg or two, these insects get on with the business of living – just like people with a disability.

In 2014, the organisation changed its name again. Moving with the times, it is now known as CPL. Each letter of its name has equal value, to highlight its mission to give people with disabilities across Queensland and northern New South Wales the freedom of **Choice**, the opportunity to chase their **Passion** and the support to live the **Life** they choose.

Chapter Four

Kindergarten And Primary School For Us!!

Dad had been taking Simon to Queensland Symphony Orchestra concerts at City Hall since he was three, as he really enjoyed them. With my own brand of language I asked if I could go along with them. Dad said I could when I was older and able to sit for longer in my stroller. When I was about four, I went to my first concert and had a wonderful time. Chris, on the other hand, was very happy doing his own thing, playing with good old Mother Nature or quietly organising his toy soldiers.

About that time my brothers and I started a really strange habit of dashing up to the end of the street and racing home again. Simon and Chris' little legs were pumping as they ran with me in the stroller. I thought that this was a great game! They were quite sturdy and well built for their ages, thanks to Mum's great cooking. Two doors up from our place we would slow down to catch our breath and walk home because we didn't want our parents to get wind of what we were doing, when we had been expressly told not to.

When Simon had his fourth birthday, Mum started asking around the neighbourhood to find a good kindergarten for my brothers. She discovered a very good kindergarten just down the road from our place.

The teacher in charge, Miss Newman, was a rather charming old lady who loved young children and being in their company. Upon our arrival she greeted us warmly with welcoming arms. This time I decided not to be my normal noisy self as I knew that this was an appointment concerning my brothers for a change.

Seeing I was disabled, Miss Newman asked what kind of condition I had. Mum replied, "Cerebral palsy, which was caused by a lack of oxygen at birth". Miss Newman commented that it was never too early for children to be aware that there are some children with special needs. Mum readily agreed with her and told her how much I enjoyed playing with my brothers and the neighbours from next door. Both agreed that it was regrettable that I would have to go to another kindergarten elsewhere in Brisbane.

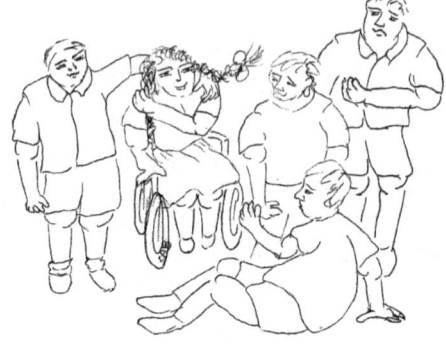

In those days there was a policy of separating disabled children from other kids. My family did not agree with this approach, so I played a lot more with other children in the neighbourhood than would otherwise be the case.

The kindergarten run by Miss Newman and a couple of helpers was located in an old family home and catered for about 25 children, plus one extra. I was the extra one because Mum and I were welcome there anytime. Most afternoons we arrived half an hour before we were due to collect my brothers. Thanks to Miss Newman's encouragement, the children were quite receptive and included me in their games.

I just loved being with other children, instead of just having Mum around as she cared for my daily needs. This really helped me get along with other people.

However, I remember a boy who was a year older than Simon, but rarely spoke to him. One day, he decided to share a game of blocks with Simon. While they were playing he asked, "Why does your mother even bother bringing your kid sister down here half an hour early every day? You know with that brain of hers, there's no way she'll get any better anyway."

As he was talking, you could almost see the steam coming out of Simon's ears. I think that he was ready to belt this kid until Miss Newman, who overheard what had been said, yelled as she raced toward her office, "Billy, meet me in my office NOW, Simon everything will be all right, just hold on".

Apparently Billy had told his parents about my mother regularly taking me to the kindergarten. Their remarks were typical of the lack of awareness and ignorance of the day. There was a lot of unfounded fear about the disabled as well. Billy tried to explain to his parents that I was different but they would not hear of it. The end result was Miss Newman instructing Billy to march out and say he was "really sorry" to Simon.

In 1959, Simon started school at Graceville State School. These buildings were built in late 1920s, so they were pretty old and were painted in a rusty bright red colour, which Mum said was left over from the war effort.

Simon was a keen learner and settled in straight away. He decided to do his reading homework every day straight after afternoon tea. Even at the age of six, Simon had great plans for his future. Right from the word go he wanted to be a musician. During the May holidays he told our parents that he would love to start learning the piano. He had seen a sign outside Graceville Catholic School, 'Music lessons here'. My parents didn't really like the idea of sending him there even for an hour a week because Mum had heard that the nuns could be quite cruel, even to small boys. Dad and Mum tried to tell him this, but he totally refused to listen. So it was that Simon began taking piano lessons and so it was that Dad and Mum were right.

My memory is that the piano room was in an old run-down convent building. I always felt this building had a pretty grim atmosphere when we went in there. Simon was always very determined and he continued having piano lessons in that awful place for another three years. Little did we know that he would grow up to travel the world as a renowned violist, as well as a devoted family man. He is also a very kind brother and takes the welfare of his family members quite seriously.

When it was Chris' turn to start his education it was an entirely different matter. Chris just wanted to continue doing things with his hands, and playing with his toy soldiers all day in kindergarten. The thought of starting his formal education did not inspire him, he was just not interested in classroom learning but he knew that he had to do it. After quite a bit of complaining he resigned himself to starting school. At the beginning of 1960, he joined his brother walking the corridors of Graceville State School. Although Chris' favourite subject was lunchtime, he was a good student for the subjects he didn't mind, like English and reading. From the first afternoon after school he diligently did his reading homework. But when it came to mathematics, or the mention of, Chris would just go to dust and want to run out of the room.

By the time I was four-and-a-half, Mum had been taking me down to New Farm for treatment for three years. One day the social worker told her there was a kindergarten on the site, and it would be good for me to make friends with other children with disabilities for a change.

This pleased my mother because she knew I would soon have to accept that I would have to attend a special class for cerebral palsy children.

So it was agreed that I would start going to kindergarten by bus within four weeks. I was quite pleased about this but at the same time I knew that I would really miss the other children at Miss Newman's kindergarten. Now that my two brothers were gone all day, I wanted a place where I could go for the entire day. My first impression of kindy was really cool and I felt really proud of myself.

By lunch on my first day I had already made a good friend, and remember thinking just how disabled Vicky was. I was taken aback that she had no use of her arms and legs. Apart from the fact we all were disabled in some way or other, we were just like any other pack of children who just played around all day.

And the kindergarten was run along the same lines as any other early learning centre, except for two things – very tired children and therapies.

Obviously, allowances had to be made for the fact that as very young children we found it tiring having to travel from our homes to New Farm; in some cases this could take up to two hours. So, in the afternoon, we were forced to have a nap, but sleeping was never a strong point of mine.

The other vital consideration was the various weekly therapies we had to 'endure'. This is the correct description because when you are that young, you don't fully understand the whole impact of your disability, and the role therapists play in your life. This is a real pity because you only have 18 years before your muscles tighten up for good. So if you don't work as hard as you can in therapy when you are a child, it makes the rest of your life much harder.

I remember being told off all the time for sitting the wrong way when I was a little girl. I really liked sitting in a low crouch with my knees wide and my bottom on the ground. This was very comfy, although everybody told me I mustn't because it could dislocate my hips. My physio used to shout at me about it, and my parents too, and although I tried not to, sometimes I just forgot.

For two years before I started school I went regularly to a speech therapist in South Brisbane. She was a very pleasant older woman with a beautiful complexion, plus she was a very good therapist, and she would give me an extremely colourful rag doll during treatment that I liked very much. I have no doubt that this therapy led to me having the ability to express myself and speak much more fluently throughout my life.

1961 was the year I started at the State School for Spastic Children, eight classrooms in the same grounds as the kindergarten, with about 80 kids. The headmistress, Miss Hilda Paul, had spent time in Birmingham, England at Carlson House School for children with cerebral palsy. The guidance officer had an office in the school as well, we saw him twice a year so that we could talk over any problems. There was a small fleet of buses that provided much needed transport to and from school, taking a great burden from families.

My first grade teacher Miss Walker was a short, plump, English lady who always wore a smile and was very kind. She was pretty tough but understanding. When we were naughty she would punish us so we all showed her total respect. She was an excellent teacher and always treated us like 'normal' kids.

Although a huge amount of water has gone under the bridge since then, I can remember starting school very well. The first thing I recall is someone pushing my tiny old wooden wheelchair down to a classroom right at the end of the corridor. I was crying quite a lot because I didn't know anyone, or what the teachers expected of me, and I felt scared.

At the same time, I felt really excited that I was starting my formal education. Miss Walker arranged us in groups of three according to our ability. After morning tea she introduced the first girl in my group, seeing as I was still a bit upset. Her name was Patricia Wain, Patty for short, and she was a year older than me. Along with 30 other children she had to stay in the hostel during term time because her parents lived outside Toowoomba, more than 100 km west of Brisbane. She was to become my first lifelong friend. When Miss Walker put our two little wooden desks together we started talking and never stopped.

Then I heard a voice coming from a physiotherapy mat, "My name is Bruce, it's good to meet you Margaret". The boy on the mat had been in the Royal Brisbane Hospital before Christmas for a hip operation.

Fifty years ago treatment and therapy was not as advanced as it is today. The only choice physiotherapists had for children with tight muscles was to put them in plaster so that they could move and walk better. This was a very long and often painful process for the child. Thankfully, I didn't have tight leg muscles, so I avoided the horror of going into plaster.

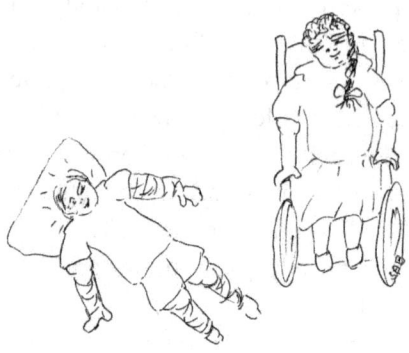

Up to that point I had not seen anyone who found it hard to move around before, except my kindergarten friend Vicky. In those days I had free movement in all four limbs. My biggest problem was that I involuntarily hit people if they were too close to me.

When I turned around and saw Bruce lying there unable to move at all something triggered inside my brain. My mind was racing like wildfire and, without moving my lips, I said to myself, "Welcome to the real world. This is the darker side of my life". Because of my disability, I would see a lot more pain and suffering in my lifetime than a non disabled person would.

When I started school my occupational therapist decided I would attend the hostel dining room five days a week to begin feeding myself. She was quite pleasantly plump and had a very friendly face. Because her attitude was always to try to help people I called her 'Mrs Lovey' and I loved her throughout my childhood years.

Now for a young girl with very protective parents, this was a confronting prospect. At home I pretty much fed myself, with a little bit of support. They knew when I was mucking around, like every time we had oxtail, which Dad loved but I hated. At those meals I would always get into trouble.

The problem was, at five-and-a-half, I still had not developed a taste for food. The only things I ate easily and happily were egg flips, bananas and some vegetables. Not only did I not like food but especially the stuff they served at school!

I can still remember my first day in the dining room, the therapist showing me how she wanted me to feed myself. This I could do until just a few years ago. So I had a go at it but the food went everywhere and I didn't like what I was being asked to eat. When she came back to check on me, it was obvious I could do it myself but was not impressed with institutional food. So she gave me a really big hug and told me just how proud of me she was.

During the first week of school the physiotherapy department sent home a letter seeking permission to give me extra physio during religious education throughout the school year. My parents said 'Yes' without even asking me because they wanted me to have as much therapy as possible.

It was these sorts of decisions that, at times, made me feel resentful towards them. Nevertheless I will always be grateful to my parents for making this decision, even though I was very curious about religion at the time. In retrospect, if I didn't have the extra physio as a child, I wouldn't have built up my muscles so I could control my movements so well.

I've had a bit of a mixed view on religion at different times of my life. Sometimes I took the view that religious education could wait until I was much older. Dad always told us that as a boy, he and his brother John had to go church two or three times every Sunday. When Dad married Mum, he decided to be a non-believer. Consequently, there were no Christian beliefs taught in our house and it was certain that neither Mum nor Dad would have felt I was special in God's eyes.

During the early years there were quite a lot of chances for me to embrace religion at school. Why? Because physio was boring and I was still curious to know what religion was all about. I soon formed the view there was a god of some form or other. I remember as a child wondering whether various people I saw as being important were a human type of god. I also felt that this god could have been close to me. This human god could be quite kind to me, but at other times he or she would treat me entirely differently. Also I had another concept of god, one high up in the heavens. Either way, something told me that this greater being could comfort me throughout my life. My parents, as indeed did I, really hated god-fearing people who would come up to me in my stroller, pat me on the head and tell me "God wanted this". To this day, I still cannot see this as anything other than condescending!

As life would have it, in my 40s I found comfort in religion to help me through a very difficult time when I was having problems with my back and trying to adjust to being much less mobile.

Chapter Five

The Early 60s

Our early childhood years were an important time for me personally, as well as the whole family. For one thing, we decided to buy a four-bedroom beach house at Labrador in the same Gold Coast street that Dad's parents lived. That was frightening! As you have probably already worked out, they were forbidding people.

I remember this beach house so well. One particular memory was a time we were driving down the long easement from the house on our way home. All three of us must have been tired because we were arguing over a toy, and Mum got really cross with us. At this point I felt so angry with my mother that I felt the need to defend the three of us. So without another thought I opened my mouth and said in a clear voice, "Shut up, Mrs Oswell!"

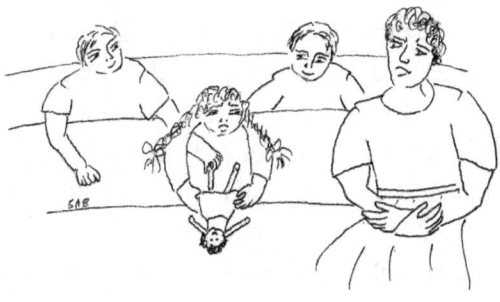

The whole car went deathly silent for a few minutes until Mum said to me, "Margaret, did I hear you talking in our language, not in your language!! You are wonderful, now you have almost taught yourself to speak English." The mood in the car turned from disbelief to jovial humour, as everybody laughed.

For the duration of our early primary schooling we escaped down to the coast most weekends, to get away from the pressure of school and living in Brisbane. Sometimes we would take my school friend Patty with us and she loved breaking out of the hostel for a whole two days. Apart from Dad and Mum both having their parents living there, this holiday house was good for my health. As a youngster, I often had a cold. Every month or so, until I was seven, I would get sick and have to stay home for a week.

I can still remember having whooping cough at the age of four. It starts with a sore throat and a general feeling of being unwell, then turns into weeks of uncontrollable gasping coughs. Of course I was quarantined at home because it's highly-infectious and can be fatal for young children. That's why babies are immunised against whooping cough these days.

For me, growing up in the 60s as a girl who just happened to be disabled, I went about my life just like any other youngster would live out her childhood, living with my family at Chelmer in the western suburbs of Brisbane.

I had the good fortune to have parents who made a point of taking me out into the community, which was rare at the time. I would go out with Dad on Saturday morning. Mostly we would go to hardware stores which, strangely, I really enjoyed and I had a real fascination with tools, particularly the hammers. And sometimes on Sunday we would go out as a whole family, just like any other household.

In 1963 it was announced that our headmistress Miss Paul had resigned to get married. When we heard this, we were all completely shocked because it never occurred to us that she would ever leave.

My parents were very disappointed that she left so suddenly. Being their only daughter, they were proud of my school achievements and they wanted to keep changes to a minimum.

Although she had three young children at home, Mum was still very interested in what was going on in the education world and she often talked to Mr Cliff, our guidance officer, when she helped as a feeding and toileting mother on the school veranda.

My next headmaster was a very jolly bloke called Mr Geoffrey Swan who was more an ally to everybody, rather than the head of a school. Looking on this era of my life yes, he was a great friend to us all and we all warmed to him and really loved him. He and his wife Doris became great family friends of ours. I well remember having tea with them in their beautiful old Gothic house. However, the head of school is there to provide leadership, so he didn't seem to have a lot of time left to give us emotional support. Of course I had unwavering support from Mum and the rest of my family, but I do feel we missed out a bit on this level at school as we were growing up.

Straight away Mr Swan took one look at the school's curriculum and made changes. It was very structured and only really suited the most intelligent students who were fortunate enough to cope with the amount of schoolwork. While I coped quite well, being one of the bright students, I found the work and travel plus five therapy sessions every week, as well as putting up with my two brothers, a real handful.

For everyone's benefit Mr Swan moved away from such a structured curriculum to one where the teachers and other staff grouped the children according to their development and intelligence. This system was based upon an interdisciplinary study by researchers from a number of different fields. Later, in 1967, Geoffrey Swan won a Churchill Fellowship overseas, so that he could study these teaching techniques for six months first hand.

Upon his return, multidisciplinary discussions were held between the various staff teams and the children for 90 minutes twice a week. The teams were made up of a teacher, occupational therapist, physiotherapist and speech therapist, and each of these professional groups took turns preparing for these sessions. If I remember correctly, we all felt a lot of pressure had been taken off us through these specialist sessions.

During these classes, I would first stand supported in a frame and then by myself, while other children were in other positions. This meant we couldn't work at our desks but our teachers kept us busy. The idea was to keep bodies moving and make our muscles stronger by reducing the time we were sitting inactive. One year we had a series of wonderful debates during this no-desk time, on things like 'Was God real' and 'Who believed in UFOs'. There was a lot of heated argument between teams. One time a man even fell though the ceiling during our debate... but I don't think we caused it!

I should explain that he was an electrician working up in the roof. When he put his foot in the wrong place, a ceiling panel collapsed under his weight and down he came.

Having a father who was head of a rather large architecture practice meant that we all had some responsibility to the firm. Every two or three months, Dad would bring home a client whom he wanted to impress. In most cases he was having trouble gaining that particular client's work. On these nights we were allowed to eat in our formal dining room and this was a great privilege, so we knew we had to be good.

You knew it, the three of us were given a real lecture by both Dad and Mum about how we were to behave – such as being polite and my brothers watching their table manners. Then they turned to me and together they would say, "Margaret, you know the drill only too well! Your father will be feeding you so you must be very careful how you eat and *don't forget to use your towel after every mouthful. Or else!*" My parents were smiling as they reminded me to do this. I replied, "You know I will do this for you both".

For a week before this big occasion, Mum would get out her many recipe books and discuss with Dad and us what she would cook for this very important guest. After the menu was decided she was happy until the day before the dinner party, when she would do all the grocery shopping. On the day of the banquet Mum and I would start in the kitchen mid-afternoon and work steadily until it was time to get me dressed.

About this time, Dad was sitting in the drawing office talking to one of his draftsman and he saw just how cramped the room was becoming. During the rest of that week he kept noticing that the rest of the office was getting too confined. He discussed this situation with a few of his employees, and they all agreed with him, the office was really becoming quite overcrowded and uncomfortable to work in. Some of them went as far as to say that he needed to think of moving to a bigger office somewhere else in the city.

That night, we were so excited when he told us his news that F.B. Oswell & Associates had so much work coming in, the whole office had to move to a more suitable location. All four of us lined up to give him a big kiss to congratulate him. However within the next few minutes, we three kids wished to take that big kiss back.

What he said then meant he did not deserve the kiss in our eyes. And that was, "During the time I am looking for a new office, we might only go down to the coast once a fortnight, if this is okay with you, Glen?"

At that moment all three of us were thinking of that beautiful new sandpit Dad had just finished building us. Now we could only use it once a fortnight. Believe me we were not happy to say the least. My brothers stormed out of the room, and I very quickly hopped off my chair and very noisily crawled out of the room too, without looking at either Mum or Dad.

When we all cooled down, we decided that this was very important to our father and to the future of the company as well; in turn this meant our future, especially mine. After an hour we decided to reappear in order of our ages. Mum saw us first and remarked, "Well, it's about time you three calmed down. We know you're all bitterly disappointed about this decision. But you are now old enough to think about your future and what your father's work means to you". She was right and we were very happy to agree with her.

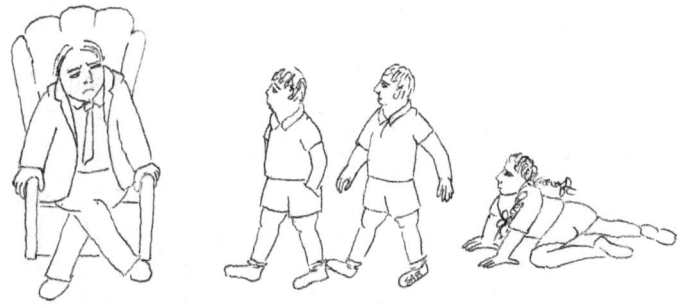

That Friday night we went down the coast to see both our grandparents, seeing that we agreed to start our search for Dad's new office the next weekend. Come Saturday morning we all happily gathered around our old kitchen table, looking through newspaper advertisements for a suitable office space. There was an office in the eastern suburbs, but Dad didn't particularly want his new premises to be there. It was better for the company to be in the central business district and more practical when he, or his employees, had to go out and inspect different sites.

These small details didn't worry us, we just wanted to go out somewhere. So after a while Mum said, "Kids, get in the car. Marg, I will walk you so that you don't get too dirty before we leave". Often Dad would just drive us around checking out places he had marked in the newspaper without really knowing where we were going, but we knew that we were going somewhere! It was a hobby of ours.

The search for a new office was long and hard. It took over three months, but when we discovered the right office we all knew it straight away. On this particular Sunday morning we were all about to give up any hope of finding the right place. Dad was reading the newspaper and taking a break from it all when this advertisement found us.

Even the location of this building was in a prime location because it was in Spring Hill, close to the heart of Brisbane. One of the oldest suburbs in the city, some of the houses dated back to the 1870s. Even today, the area has an interesting assortment of old buildings mingled with modern structures.

"Let's go, this one looks really hopeful," I said. It didn't take long from home to reach the centre of the city. We had driven through Spring Hill countless times but had not taken much notice of it. Today we were all much more interested in the area, seeing as we might be buying into it and be able to resume our regular trips to our beloved Gold Coast house and, of course, that new sand pit!

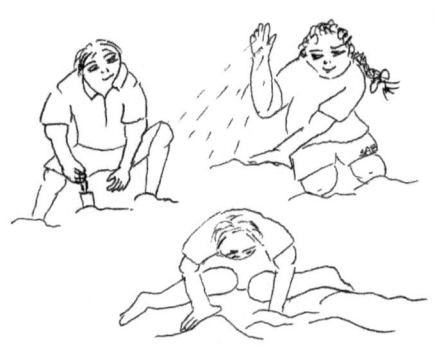

Ahead of us, on the corner of Boundary and Mills Streets, was a beautiful old white building that was quite rundown. It was an old Cobb & Co station from the early horse and cart days when Spring Hill was named for the creek that originally supplied Brisbane's drinking water. There was history all around. Back in the early settlement days, a fence was put up to keep Aborigines out of the city each night after a curfew was instituted. The track that ran along the city side of the fence was later named 'Boundary Street'.

One of the first things that caught my eye as we turned the corner was the huge backyard, which was so steep that people almost had to clamber down to reach a terrace that led into a massive room. Straight away, Dad and Mum knew that it would make a perfect drawing office. There was such a look of relief on Dad's face, in fact he was just about dancing. Another room could be used as Dad's office, where he could work on plans for his clients. And there was another small office for Pat Gibson, his fantastic secretary and a good friend to the whole family. Looking back on it, she saved our young lives on many occasions when we were naughty. Being the nice person she was, she covered up for a lot of silly things we did – like raiding the office fridge and leaving food everywhere.

Chapter Six

The Next Problem The Family Had To Face

As I remember it, the episode about to be revealed played a big role in all of our lives. Maybe it started in 1962 or 1963 but it did not culminate until August 1964. You guessed it, this whole matter was centred on me.

One morning I was going to school on the bus when the driver could hear me having an epileptic seizure, also known as a fit. While it was not a bad seizure, he pulled over for 15 minutes to make sure that I was all right. When the bus arrived at school one of the mothers helped me to change out of my wet clothes before I went down to my class. This was just a warning sign of what was to come.

Of course the school nursing sister rang Mum to tell her about the seizure. She also told her that I was quite happy to stay at school and come home on the bus as normal. Poor Mum was amazed by this; it seemed to my parents that they had just sorted out one problem when they were confronted with a new one! However, this problem was to become much bigger. Mum asked if it could happen again but nobody knew the answer. I could have a seizure again tomorrow but might not have another for two years if I was lucky.

The experts say these fits are disturbances in the normal electrical functions of the brain. I had a tonic seizure, which spreads throughout the brain, causing unconsciousness and twitching in the arms and legs. Other characteristics are biting the tongue and loss of bladder control, as I experienced on the bus.

For about four months I was free from any seizures. Then, once again, I was going to school on the bus when I had my second episode. The sister thought there was something in the bus travel that could be causing them. Mum was stunned as I loved school and there were never any worries about me wanting to go. It was decided I would continue taking the bus to school for the time being.

Over the next 12 to 18 months, the seizures occurred more often and became more severe. Instead of having tonic seizures, I was beginning to have fits called 'tonic clonic', also known as Grand Mal, which spread over both hemispheres of the brain at the same time. I would be unconscious, sometimes for 10 minutes or more, which was rather dangerous. Now my whole body, including my arms and legs, would convulse violently. The worst and most dangerous thing was that my tongue would block my airway. This of course meant that I could not get any oxygen and, as a result, I turned bright blue. A bit like something out of Avatar!

The first few times I had this kind of seizure the bus driver brought me out of it but each time it was becoming more difficult without medical help. Afterwards I would be dazed and tired. When we arrived at New Farm there was an oxygen tank in the nurse's office to help me recover. It was black, and would really frighten me.

By now my parents were apprehensive about what would happen if I needed immediate medical assistance. One night they had yet another discussion about the subject, and Mum decided to start driving me to school because she felt I would be more comfortable in a car rather than on the bus.

Dad agreed, however one point concerned him - Mum driving from our suburb on the other side of town to New Farm 10 times a week, on top of all her other duties. He felt it would get terribly tiring for her.

Then I had a seizure in the classroom and another one before I went to bed one night. Because of these latest episodes, Mum was becoming a bit afraid of the possibility of me taking a huge fit while I was in the car with her, but she still went through with the idea. For about five months, I didn't have any problems, then I had a tiny one.

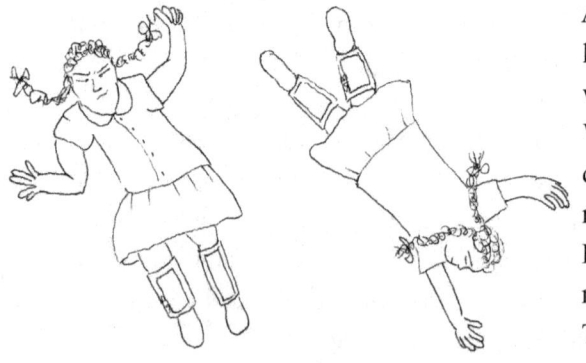

A fortnight later it happened. What we feared most. While we were driving through a really busy part of Brisbane, I had a massive seizure. This one was so big that after 10 minutes I was showing no signs of coming out of it like I usually did. Poor Mum! She was always level-headed but she didn't know what to do. There was no choice but to call the ambulance.

Even after being given first aid, I still did not come out of my seizure. So, after half an hour of holding up the traffic, I had my first trip to hospital. Of course, Mum came with me and, by this time, she'd rung Dad, who met us there.

I spent a week in the Royal Brisbane Children's Hospital only five kilometres from where the incident took place. I remember being in the second ward (the little girls' ward). In one of the beds there was a girl whose bones were so brittle they would break every time her parents picked her up to give her a hug. When I saw that, it made me feel so sorry for her. I thought to myself, I might have cerebral palsy, but her parents cannot even give her a big cuddle when she needs one.

During the week the doctors did a series of tests by putting a very strange hat on my head and attaching some wires to it. This was so they could record my brain waves and determine for sure the type of epileptic fits I was experiencing. Mum made a point of being with me when I had these tests, because I was still only eight years old.

As always, my family were there for me. Mum would come and spend most of the day, then return late in the afternoon with my brothers. Dad would come and see me when he finished work each night.

My first stay in hospital, the first of many, was all right. On the seventh day I was allowed to go home, provided that I went to a see a neurologist, a specialist in brain disorders and the nervous system.

All of these events are what led to the August 1964 culmination of us moving house.

Chapter Seven

Dad's Solution To The Whole Problem

It felt really good to be home in my own environment once more, especially knowing the doctors would find a way of controlling my fits.

The neurologist we saw the next day looked at all the test results from the hospital, and then examined me. She decided to put me on anti-convulsant drugs used to control most epileptic fits. There are many of these drugs on the market. The type a doctor prescribes depends on things like age, overall health and medical history as well as the frequency and severity of the seizures.

Dilantin, or Phenytoin Sodium, was the drug the doctor prescribed me, and it is well-known for being effective in preventing seizures. I remember these slow-release orange and white capsules well because Dad used to tease me about the colour of them all the time. Maybe they reminded him of the many household fires they lit in Victoria to keep warm when he was a boy.

I still take anti-convulsant medication to this day, and haven't had a seizure in years.

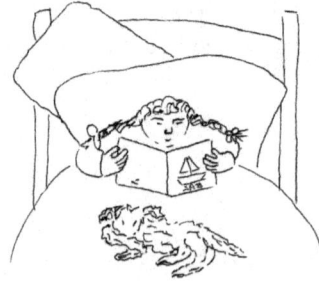

The doctor wanted me to have another week off school, so that the drugs would have a chance to get into my system. I was not pleased about this at all! But after my usual huff and pout, I knew why it had to be. As Dad pointed out, Mum was really tired and had not recovered from the shock of my large seizure. She was afraid of the mere thought of driving me to New Farm. After a period of grace the drugs entered my system. Meanwhile Dad worked in secret on his solution to the whole problem.

Sometimes I wonder what else he kept secret and for how long! When Mum raised her concerns about taking me to school, he just replied by saying, "Well Glen, don't be too concerned about it. Now the Dilantin is in her system, Marg should be all right to go to school on the bus until we can arrange something else."

It was about this time that Dad started disappearing from the office. He didn't tell any of his staff where he was going and nobody knew when he would be back. He could not have been spending all this time with his best clients.

No, he was using his knowledge of buildings to find a suitable cheap old house close to school where a family of five people could live quite comfortably. Somehow Dad heard of an auction sale of a terribly old house, which for the last two years had been used as a builder's warehouse and labourers' tearoom, while they were constructing the first high-rise in New Farm.

Believe me, it was a real mess. What became my bath even had tea and coffee poured down the drain. The rest of house was a complete eyesore, full of gaping holes and other damage. The labourers must have assumed that the house would be demolished after they had finished with it, because they shifted all the dirt from the site into what was to become our new place.

But Dad, with his practised eye, could visualise what could be done with this poor, gentle old house, with a little elbow grease and some extensive repairs.

While he went to the auction with the view of buying a new family home to live in, the rest of the bidders were only there to pull it down because it was in such a state of disrepair.

On the day of the auction, Dad arrived home very early because he could not wait to tell us what he had done. When we heard the door open and saw him come in, we could hardly believe it. Something was obviously up! It was Mum who spoke first, "What are you doing home at this hour? Are you sick?"

"No, I'm not, in fact I am the opposite. I have found the solution to our problem of how Marg will get to school in future, in case she starts taking seizures on the bus once more. Today, I went to an auction sale and bought a house in New Farm that is only 500 metres from the Spastic Centre."

Mum yelled, "Just why did you do that without consulting me first?" To this, Dad shouted back in a louder voice, "And you would have talked me out of it! Besides I didn't know if I would get an opportunity to buy it".

Mum thought about this and conceded, "Frank, I've decided to reserve judgement about the house until we see it for ourselves".

We decided to wake up early on Saturday morning and inspect the old house. Mum helped me get ready, seeing we were both very eager, but what greeted us at 41 Griffith Street was not a pretty sight, believe you me. In fact poor Mum just threw her hands in the air in complete and utter horror and said loudly, "You call this a house, I call it a heap of junk!"

The front door had been kicked in by the builders. The view which greeted us was a two metre layer of filthy black dirt, spread all over the place so we could not see the other wall of the house.

Dad was the first person to break the silence that came upon the family as we looked at all that muck. In his defence he said, "I know what you are thinking but with the necessary repairs and my knowledge of building structure, I can remodel this house quite easily."

"You have a good point there," said Mum smiling and her mood lighter. "Let's keep walking through the house and see what actually needs to be done and how much it will cost."

"Marg, watch your step," she said as I tightened my grip on Dad's wrist. "There is junk all over all the place so please be very careful not to fall over."

As we walked through the house it seemed that Dad was right after all. We decided it was not the bomb site we first thought it was. And it was right on the Brisbane River.

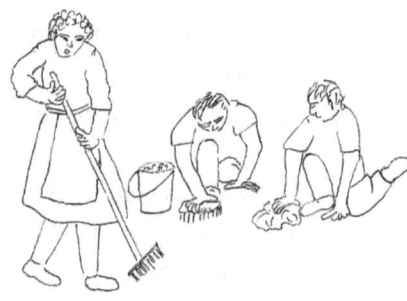

Despite the mess, the house was indeed structurally sound. It just needed a big dose of tender loving care from us all. These were Mum's favourite words for every situation in life. We began by sweeping the house, probably for the first time in years. Brooms flew in every direction as our excitement soared, along with the dust.

As the years of dirt and grime were slowly washed away, I found a corner in what became our living room, where I watched enthralled the changes to the old house. On the way home, there were five exhausted bodies in the car, but at the same time, we were five really happy bodies with a new house.

Good old Dad was so right when he said it would be a wonderful house for children to grow up in. This house meant such a lot to me and my mobility. It was our home for 20 years. Looking back, it was where I spent most of the years when I could move freely and easily.

Obviously freedom of movement was important for me, and my parents did everything they could to progress my physical development. When I was in my early teens, the five of us would pack up the car on Boxing Day each year and head westwards along any roads we wanted to travel. Mum and Dad had one very strict rule on these trips, which was that I was to throw away my boots and irons for a whole week. This was real freedom and I did it with great joy. Between school and therapy, I was very tired by Christmas time and needed a complete break that was a real adventure.

Chapter Eight

Moving Into Our New Home

On Monday morning, when Dad had time between his normal office work, he started ringing around various tradesmen to get quotes and find out how soon they could start work. The first job was to find some labour to remove the endless mountain of dirt from upstairs.

After many phone calls, Dad found a building firm who could fix the structural damage in about two weeks at a reasonable price. They were not able to start the job sooner because of commitments on other building sites. Because all the electrical wiring had been damaged by the builders prior to us buying the house, Dad had an electrician completely rewire the whole place, which took a further three weeks. This meant that we could not move in until the August holidays. Mum pointed out that this was a good time to move. It gave us a bit of extra time to complete this whole change, then in the second week we three kids could start exploring our new neighbourhood in our own time, which she knew we would!

Over the next week Mum asked us to begin thinking about what toys and other things we wanted to take with us, and what could be thrown out. Immediately I thought of my large rag doll collection, and knew I had to take them because I could not survive without them. At that time my favourite rag doll was one called 'Harry the horse'. He was adorable, shaped like a tiny seahorse and could fit into my right hand.

All three of us were excited about the coming adventure. However, we all felt very sad about leaving our first home and our neighbours. They had been good neighbours and we had grown to know them well.

When I was growing up, there were not many times I considered myself more fortunate than my two brothers but, in this case, I did. This time it worked in my favour as I did not have to change schools or leave all my friends behind as the boys did, in fact I could have more time with my friends. When Mum told my two brothers that she was going to enrol them at New Farm State School she got two very different reactions. Simon always had a joyful expression on his face when there was talk of school. Chris was completely different in his reactions. He just looked at Mum with a really sad expression on his face as if to say, "Do I have to go to school? Why can't I have the term off, please!"

Mum reassured Chris that when it came time to change schools, she would go with him. Then he too was very excited to be starting at New Farm State School.

To Simon this move meant relief from being punished continually by the nuns at Graceville convent during his piano lessons. From all accounts the nuns at Fortitude Valley were really cool and more progressive. Dad and Mum thought that they would be kinder to both my brothers, as these nuns were very community minded. We soon found they also had a great sense of humour.

Pam was another consideration in our move. Fifteen is old for a dog and she was completely blind. It was a long time before my parents had children, so Pam was the next best thing to keep them company. She was a very faithful dog to us all. Often she would sit at Mum's feet, while she fed me on the veranda.

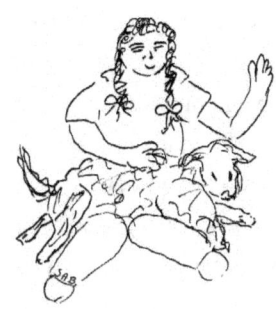

Pam was a really calm dog, when I patted her it was more like hitting because I did not have control over my hands to pat her softly. Mostly Mum would help me stroke her. We loved watching her chase Granddad's chooks. My two brothers could be horrible to Pam because they took delight in chasing her all over the backyard and I enjoyed watching them do this. Sometimes they would capture her and put her in the wheelbarrow. I would do what I could to chase her too but she would get away. I was a horror in my own way! Pam and Dad would also share time together while he was working around the house, or late at night.

All too soon it was moving time. We woke to a near perfect day. Eating our last meal at Chelmer made everybody feel very sad indeed. It was only a few minutes before the furniture truck was due to arrive. This show was going somewhere fast! I spent much of the morning hopping out of the men's way and it was soon time to lock up the house for the last time, and then follow our furniture to 41 Griffith Street. I went in Dad's car, and we took Pam too. Along the way we dropped the old house keys off at the real estate office. This meant we didn't reach the house until unloading the truck was well under way. When Dad let Pam out of the car she immediately darted around the back and we went on with the business of moving.

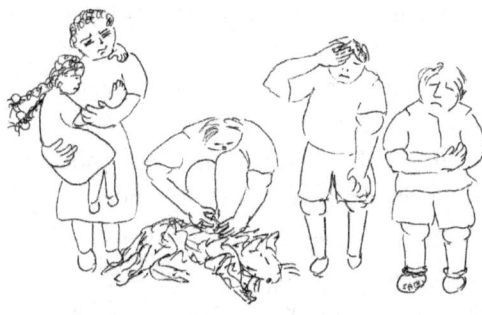

Everybody was so busy giving the men directions about what rooms the heavy pieces of furniture went in and doing a million other things. It wasn't until the moving van had left, and we sat down to a pile of sandwiches and a cup of tea, that, to our horror, we remembered the dog. It was as if a collective thought hit us, and we all yelled at once "WHERE IS SHE, WHERE'S PAM?" Because of her blindness, our greatest fear was she would not be able to find her way around and wander out onto the balcony, thinking it was the front gate. We darted about like rockets, yelling her name and expecting her to come to us, but she didn't. It was Dad and Simon who tore off in the direction of the balcony. With no sign of her, Dad was starting to breathe a sigh of relief until, to his horror, five metres below on the ancient concrete lay our much beloved pet.

On seeing this sight, Dad let out such a scream and tore down the back stairs with Simon crying in hot pursuit. Mum, Chris and I had returned to the kitchen and were alerted to this tragedy by the commotion. Mum immediately grabbed me off the floor and joined Chris as we headed downstairs as quickly as we could go. We followed Simon and Dad's voices, then the sight of Pam's crumbled body simply stopped us in our tracks. I burst into tears while Mum and Chris shook their heads in disbelief.

As we all stood over her very small body, Dad checked to see if it was worth while calling a vet, but it was too late. His head sank to his chest and he said in a very sad voice, "I am so angry with myself, I should have remembered her blindness." We all looked at each other as if to say we should have known better than to leave her by herself.

In her usual role as comforter, Mum said it was all very well to feel that way but, with the stress and busy nature of the day, our oversight was understandable. Indeed, we were equally guilty. She also remarked that not even Margaret had remembered for some reason "and, as you know, she usually remembers everything".

Chapter Nine

What We Did After That

We quickly realised nothing was left to be done for poor old Pam but, as we all knew, she had a good life. Sometimes things happen for a reason. She would have had a hard time finding her way around her new home, being old and blind as she was. As we moped around with heavy hearts, Pam was already sniffing around in all the corners of heaven.

It was mid-afternoon by now and our new house looked like a world war had hit it. Everybody, apart from Dad who stayed downstairs to bury Pam's body somewhere in the overgrown wilds of the garden, headed upstairs again to begin the task ahead of us.

As he was the eldest, Simon was given a bedroom in one corner of the house, with space to keep all his music and other things. Chris and I shared a bedroom space, separated by our cupboards. While this idea worked well, it was never intended to be permanent. Dad had already been up into the roof and knew attic bedrooms could be build sometime in the future. As it was, we both had just enough room and the arrangement stayed in placed for several years.

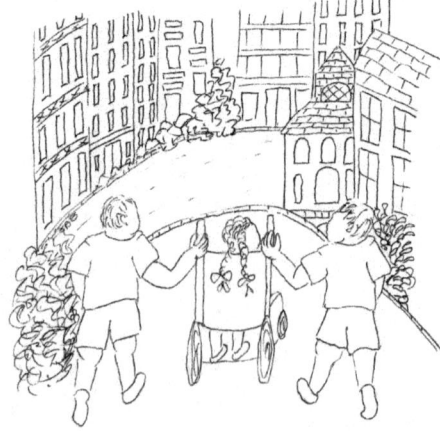

Of course, Mum and Dad had the master bedroom with an adjoining bathroom that I also used. When I was a child, and right up to my early 40s, I found it very easy to get into a bath myself and I really enjoyed them. It's a shame that the sort of bath I could wheel myself into nowadays is much too big for an ordinary house.

On that first day we didn't do much else except get our new house ready so we could go to bed for the night. Although we were feeling sad about what happened to Pam, we all had a good feeling that this house would be our home for many years to come. After a simple dinner of fish and chips with salad, which we all enjoyed, we three decided to start exploring our new district. We wanted to find out how many cool kids lived in our street.

It was only two or three days before one of our neighbours came down to introduce herself. Mum had just finished washing the breakfast dishes when she answered a knock at the door. There was a casually dressed woman who we all fell in love with straight away. She was New Farm's number one gossip but a very kind gossip, if you were careful to watch your P's and Q's, and she would do anything for you.

"Welcome to the district, my name is Mrs Luke, and I live four doors up, with my husband Arthur and my two boys Geoffrey and Russell. Would you like to come up to my place to have a cup of coffee this morning?"

Mum willingly agreed. Over the next week or two, Mrs Luke started turning up at our place at 4 o'clock every afternoon for a cup of coffee and a chat. This chat was more often than not very one-sided because she liked to hold the floor and Mum and I couldn't get a word in edge ways. After a fortnight of Mrs Luke coming down to see us every day at the same time we realised that she was probably a very lonely person.

Mrs Luke wasn't the only character in our street at New Farm. Our nearest neighbours Maisy and Vince were characters of a different kind and had a big influence on the family. They were retired publicans from the Port Office Hotel, in downtown Brisbane—a very popular watering hole in the early days of the city. Coming from this background they were quite fascinating people and we really loved listening to them talk about their hotel career, and living above a pub.

Besides this they had a Morton Bay cruiser, called *Maisvin* moored to a jetty at the bottom of their garden. Being children, we had never been on a big boat like this before so were keen to give it a go.

It was not long before Mum took us to visit Maisy and Vince so we could ask them ourselves. At that time Vince was the commander of the 18 Footers Yacht Club, which was in the Hamilton reach of the Brisbane River, downstream of New Farm. Mum explained we were all very interested in looking at their boat, if they didn't mind us asking.

Both of them immediately invited us to look over the boat and have morning tea on board, and a date was decided on the spot. Mum, who hated boats, decided she would not go, but Dad and I and the boys were very excited at the prospect.

It was all so different to Chelmer. Mum and Dad once told me it took about 20 years for the neighbours there to even say "HELLO". The primary reason for this was they were living in a caravan when they first moved there, while building our first house in stages. All in all I have an idea it took four years to finish the whole house so they were quite preoccupied. Dad always said that building was in his heart and I tend to agree with him. Here at this new house the neighbours were interested to get to know us and my parents were pleasantly surprised that anyone would make the effort.

Maisvin was built in the old style with her sides well above her decks. Although she had a few years on her, she was still a very stylish and comfortable boat because the owners poured a lot of love into her.

Sometimes my brothers, Dad and I would go out on the boat and watch the first sort of yacht racing we had ever seen. Back then the Brisbane River was not nearly as polluted as it is today, it was so clear on occasion that we could see right down to the bottom. On one of those days we were looking over the side into the water and we saw a huge lung fish. It was such an amazing sight, one memory I shall never forget from my childhood. These strange-looking fish have long since disappeared from the now-murky Brisbane River.

For three years we saw Maisy and Vince tending their beautiful garden and *Maisvin*. They were perfect neighbours, except Mum always had to allow three hours to go to their place; because Maisy poured a mean gin. It took all that time for poor Mum to drink a glass because it was so potent.

Simon and Vince had become the best of mates; they spent a lot of time together, and we weren't far behind. Then for a while we hardly saw either Maisy or Vince around the garden or boat. Simon was growing concerned that our friend's heart was playing up. So he alerted Mum and Dad and they went in to find out.

Sure enough Simon was right! Vince told them he was under doctor's orders to rest as much as possible as his ticker was not so good. As soon as

Simon heard about this he took it upon himself to give Vince and Maisy two hours a week, so that he could help them around their garden and boat.

Living on the river and getting to know Vince and Maisy opened up a whole new avenue of adventure for Dad and the boys, as well as Mum and I. They all became keen yachtsmen and sailed and raced a succession of boats together, and with friends, for quite a few years.

Dad had already introduced Simon and Chris to the joys of sailing when he bought them a little Sabot class training yacht down on the Gold Coast a couple of years before, but once we moved to New Farm they all became much more serious and competitive. Little did we know that these early weekend experiences would lead to a boating career for Chris.

Too soon, our settling-in week was over, and Chris and Simon had to front up to their new school. Being the horrible sister that I was, I poked fun at them, instead of supporting them, seeing that I didn't have to change schools. On the Monday morning, Mum took me to school, then enrolled Simon, who just took himself down to his classroom to meet his teacher. Chris lacked the confidence to do this but went down to his classroom quite willingly with Mum. He was maturing and seemed to be applying himself to his schooling much better. This was something we were all really proud of.

My teacher at the time was the first overseas teacher I came across. This was Miss Pamela Hatch, a young Englishwoman with a funny accent and jet black hair, who was always full of joy. By the second year of school I had gained enough from physiotherapy to venture from my wooden wheelchair to a walking frame. She would look especially tense whenever I walked into the classroom, and she was right to be tense because some days I would fall over six or seven times. Often I would laugh when I did this but there were also times when I would fall backwards and hit my head, which made me cry.

My parents were always encouraging me to take my education seriously, so this year I wanted to do just that. Miss Hatch was very keen to see how much I, and the other five children in my class, could learn. She was the first teacher to give me an insight into how to write an essay and instil in me a love of words. It was in this class I wrote my first story and I was very pleased with it. By this time I had been using my own typewriter for about a year, so by now my hand function was improving but my spelling was something else. It was my worst subject throughout school. Mum was always tearing her hair out over it.

Until we moved to New Farm in August 1964, Miss Hatch used to tell us what it was like living on the Brisbane River and I would imagine it as being really peaceful. When we moved, she became a close neighbour because she lived in a tiny unit under Mrs Luke's house, with a lovely lawn outside sloping down to the river.

Early in 1965, our faith in the Catholic Church was restored. The nuns who taught music at nearby St Patricks were completely different to those at Graceville. They were much more worldly as well as being understanding and caring, and were fun to be around.

The church itself was Victorian Gothic style dating back to the 1880s, with a wonderful ornate organ. Mum and I would sometimes sit in the church waiting for music lessons to finish, because it had a very quiet atmosphere about it.

Now the boys had settled into their new school, Mum and Dad decided that Chris was ready to start piano lessons. It was agreed that the sisters would give him a six-month trial to see if he had the aptitude to follow in his brother's footsteps. Unfortunately the answer was "no". As the nuns themselves put it, he didn't have an ear for music and found learning to read music sheets very difficult indeed, so he didn't want to carry on. On the other hand they felt that Simon was very talented and asked if they could start teaching him the violin, Mum was so pleased that she gave him a great big hug. When he told Dad what the nuns said about him, he got another hug. The next week he had his first violin lesson.

Every year, around September, the nuns had a concert. Even though Simon wasn't Catholic, they borrowed him for the performance. We would all go along and sit in the front row.

Now we were living on the river, Chris had developed a real interest in the Brisbane City Council ferries. One afternoon he was in the kitchen with Mum and I, and noticed one of the ferries passing a tug. Chris looked towards Mum and asked cheerfully, "What ferry is that?"

"For goodness sake, how do you think I know the difference between ferries. If you see one ferry, you might as well see all three of them. I can't tell them apart," she said.

"Mum, you're a great mother but you're really dumb. That ferry is the *Vicky Lynn*. Women are only good for cooking and kissing!" Mum stood back and stared at Chris, dumbfounded.

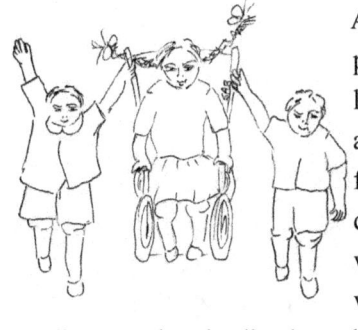

At New Farm, we kids continued our practice of racing the stroller. There was a long narrow park to the left of our place, and more often than not we would go there for a walk after school. We used to walk quite slowly until the bend in the river, then we would pick up speed, literally flying with my stroller, and took delight in startling people who lived nearby. While we were in our upper primary years, poor Mum and Dad got countless phone calls about my brothers' habit of racing in the park with their disabled sister. Well, what could my poor parents say. I was the one urging the boys to go faster and faster still.

Chapter Ten

Rebuilding The House As Life Goes On

Now we had successfully restored the upstairs level of our house, we thought we'd have a bit of a break to enjoy our new place before starting the really massive job of rebuilding downstairs. Down there we were faced with the very same thing that confronted us the first time we saw over the house, only at ground level it was even worse. I think the mountain of dirt that covered the whole of the downstairs was up to half a metre high in places. Under this mountain of terrible dark brown soil was a very thick layer of ugly stained cement, most likely from having all that dirt on it for so long.

Part of this floor was split into a level nearly a metre higher than the rest. Dad claimed this space for himself and built the most wonderful workshop of all time. The things he would create! The largest things Dad made in his workshop were two small yachts but often he would get an idea for something to make me more independent and then he would just set to work to make it. Things like fashioning a key guard on my typewriter to steady my hand on the keys. When I was young, Mum and Dad bought me an electric typewriter in the hopes I could use it for my homework because I could not write by hand and I never will. When I did try to type, my fingers would hit several keys together. Once he had thought about the problem overnight, he came up with a solution. He wondered if an iron guard across my keyboard would stop me from pressing too many letters at once. I remember him filing and filing to get it just right.

This was just one piece of the puzzle of teaching me to use a typewriter because there was another problem. My parents could clearly see that my right wrist needed to be supported somehow. This time the solution lay at the beach. One day we were playing around, filling a bag with sand...and there was the answer. Dad made a long sandbag shaped like a sausage that sat on my desk in front of the typewriter, and I still use one today with my computer.

About three weeks later, Dad was putting out the rubbish. He came upstairs and said to Mum: "I think it's time we start removing that soil from downstairs because it's driving me mad."

They decided to find a weekend handyman to help with the rebuilding effort. The boat builder who was constructing my brothers' Wright class yacht at the time knew an English bloke who was not only very skilful with his hands but trustworthy as well. So it was that Eric came into our lives. The next Saturday morning, we met one of the most delightful tradesman I ever had the pleasure of knowing. When he saw the mountain of dirt, he said in his broad Kentish accent, "Raht, ow fust jorb iss ta remuve dis orrible durt".

As much as I would have loved to help move the dirt, I was just as happy to supervise my family and join in the conversation. After quite a few weekends working from dawn to dusk shifting the dirt in wheelbarrows, we were successful in getting rid of all that dark brown soil.

That was just the beginning, for Eric and Dad then had to break up the ancient cement with their heavy hammers and clear it away. We all knew it would take many long hours of physical work and quite a few glasses of beer to achieve these results. These two workmen were well-known for doing better formwork and brick work before lunch, but what the hell!

When they had finished laying the new cement, we had a family discussion to decide what the downstairs would be used for. It was decided to have a storage area for all the sailing gear and a games room with a table tennis table, billiard table and stereo so we could play our records really loudly. We all thought this was a great idea. Nobody knew what our teenage years would bring! They say to be prepared for these years.

The staircase was really in need of repair, especially the lower steps. We all decided that this was the second major task to be done. It was here that Dad's architecture skill came into force. About that time I started to want more independence on the stairs, and not have to rely on my parents all the time. Dad, Eric and I put our heads together and devised a pulley system, using thick orange rope, 10 centimetres round, attached somewhere in the head of the stairwell. With this I could bounce on my bottom backwards from stair to stair and pull myself up the stairs, which was a lot of fun to do. All this exercise did me good, as I really had to use my legs and arms. At either end of the staircase, I would just crawl, unless one of my parents was there to walk me. This allowed me to just take myself off into the backyard when I had finished work in my room for the day.

When Simon started at Brisbane Grammar School, he quickly found it had a large music department and an orchestra. Once again he decided to change teachers to the music master at the school, so he could immerse himself in the musical activities there.

It didn't take him long to make friends at school, particularly with a new boarder, who was having a hard time adjusting to city life and being away from home for the first time ever. Simon took him under his wing and Neal has been a friend to the family ever since. He and his family lived on a cattle property just outside Emerald, in Central Queensland, about 10 hours north west of Brisbane by car.

Neal came to stay with us one long weekend, given it was too far to go home for three days. More than four decades later, he and Simon are still best mates. That is what you call a good friendship. I felt quite excited about meeting Neal because we had heard so much about him, and remembered thinking to myself, *He is what he is. A country boy at heart.* You could really see he was not comfortable with city life, and because of this, the pair of them were pretty quiet for that whole weekend. It wasn't until the second or third weekend that Neal stayed with us that we realised why he was so quiet. He was desperately homesick and missing the bush.

Meanwhile, poor Chris wasn't having much luck in his life. He wasn't enjoying school and one day in late February he came home from school with a bad headache, and a pain in the stomach. Mum told him to go to bed early and in the morning she would see if he was well enough to go to school. Next morning, he was feeling worse and the doctor was called that afternoon. He thought that it was only a virus, which all children pick up from time to time. In a few days, Chris would be running around again, which he was. For the next six weeks he was his usual 12-year-old self.

Once more he came home with a sore stomach and a bad headache, his virus had returned this time worse than ever. Again he went to bed for a day before Mum called the doctor, who said the same thing. For a period of three or four months this very same thing kept happening regularly until our mother put her foot down, and a few tests were run on him, because he was getting quite weak.

The doctor then ran a full series of blood tests, besides asking the whole family a lot of questions. Where did we, as young children spend a lot of time? And what did we like doing? Dad and Mum had to really think about this one, but then they came up with the answer. We spent a lot of time on the Gold Coast, and all three of us simply loved feeding the birds at Currumbin Bird Sanctuary. Chris would feed a dozen birds at a time, and they would be all over him. We had found the answer to the mystery virus, making him sick...some sort of bird flu! The doctor then prescribed some medicine to make him completely better.

In 1968 Chris joined his brother at Brisbane Grammar School and he really enjoyed it. He was still an outdoor boy at heart, loving his sport and playing cricket in the summer and our beloved hockey in the winter season. The school was only five minutes' walk from Dad's office, which was very handy for them with all the activities they had after school. When they were ready to come home all they had to do was take a short walk to catch a ride with Dad.

The time had come for another building project. Having only enough space in his tiny bedroom for a bed and a cupboard, there was nowhere Chris could put a desk. When Dad first looked at the house he visualised two attic bedrooms. In February, Eric and Dad rethought the idea of going up another storey, so that my brothers could live up there in peace and quiet.

During the week before Easter, when Dad didn't have much work in the office, he spent the time going around hardware stores buying materials to start building these two attic bedrooms. My favourite hobby at the time was helping Dad around the yard, or sitting in his workshop just watching him work for hours on end.

At the time I wore black or brown boots laced up to my ankles, which were pretty weak. I also had to wear short callipers until I was 16 years old. A calliper is two metal rods, one on each side of the leg, with a cross strap that fastened just below my knees. They didn't look too good but they steadied my legs really well and helped me walk. I always wore long socks to stop them hurting my legs, because they were quite tight.

My parents and I had been waiting two months for a new pair of boots to arrive. When we picked them up I was so proud of them; I somehow talked Mum into putting them on me right away because I wanted to show them to Eric. Then I simply forgot that I was wearing new boots, although I was told to be very careful of them. I was much too busy crawling around on the cement, holding pieces of wood for Dad to saw for the framework of the attic.

That night when it was bath time, Mum had to take off my ruined boots! Believe me, my mother was not a happy woman. She went right off her head at me. There was a lot of shouting in our house that night and I got a smacked bottom. This time Dad was less cross than Mum for a change, after all I had given him a lot of help during the day.

It never took my parents long to cool down after a ding-dong row with one of us. Simon and Chris had their likes and dislikes, just like everybody else who walks this earth. When Mum made Simon practise his music when he didn't want to, there was always a fight of some kind. Sometimes they would carry on for half an hour, biting each others' heads off, and other times it would only last a few minutes. Chris had his own temper because, at times, he was very stubborn and he would not give us things. His temper would only appear about once a year but, when it did, he was in a temper for days and would kick the broom that could not fight him back.

I suppose I started off with a normal temper, which could have been a bit stubborn and a bit determined. Then something happened to my temper. It took a right hand turn and did a backward dive. The only thing I can think of to account for it was when I was born and they found out I had cerebral palsy they were so concerned about the physical aspects of my disability that they somehow forgot that there was a real person growing up inside that body. A tiny person, for whom her mother and father would do anything to ease her suffering and support her welfare. Possibly their attitude and the care and non-stop support of my parents helped make my temper take this strange turn. When I was very small I don't suppose Mum and Dad understood when I was cross with people, so I ended up taking it out on them.

By the age of four, when I started talking, they knew for sure my temper had taken a backward slide. When I had one of my mood swings they would tell me off but they were not as firm as they should have been. Later, when I was in Grade 3, Mum spoke to Mr Swan about this bad behaviour and he told her not to worry about it. "With her cerebral palsy and the frustration she gets from it, it's no wonder she blows her top once a month or so," he said. Whether this advice was right or wrong, my parents accepted it and did not seek another opinion on the matter.

From the age of 10 and even into my teens I continued having temper tantrums when I couldn't get my own way, or didn't want to do what I was told. To make matters worse, when I was about 12 or 13, instead of blowing up at people I started becoming quite depressed. Over the years I've learned to keep my temper under my hat and not get depressed about things I can't change.

From memory, I think that it took three months to build the attic so it was not long before we all had new bedrooms. When Simon moved out of his room, I moved into it. It just felt so great to have my own space, I was able to have my typewriter in my room at last. I had a large wooden desk, with drawers for all my books and papers. And a big white cupboard for my clothes at the other end of the room. There was a bay window with a vast frangipani tree just outside. Whenever I could, I would curl up on the seat under the window and look up at that beautiful tree.

By this time we had been in the house a few years and I had collected even more rag dolls. I didn't want to throw them away but there was nowhere in my new bedroom to keep them. Good old Mum said I could keep them in her sewing room and play with them whenever I liked.

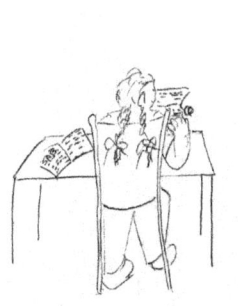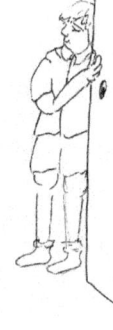One day Neal was coming down from Simon's bedroom in the attic. I was doing my homework in my room and he must have heard the sound of my typewriter keys. Without me knowing it, he stood and watched for a while. Then he must have made a noise and I turned around. "I didn't know you could type?" he said, unaware I did all my schoolwork on a

typewriter. We were already good friends but now that he actually knew just how capable I was, our friendship grew.

At the time, Simon was having violin and piano lessons in Fortitude Valley and the nun who was his teacher fell down some stairs and broke her leg, so she was no longer able to teach him. Luckily Dad knew of an architect in New Farm, who was also an accomplished violinist and teacher. His name was John Curro, from a very wealthy Italian immigrant family involved in the North Queensland sugar cane industry.

John was heavily involved in music, and Brisbane's musical scene, so much so he established the Queensland Youth Orchestra, which Simon joined. Then he started to have private lessons from John, who became his new mentor.

When John first heard Simon play the piano and violin, he was astonished at what he was hearing. In fact it was John who first told Simon how talented he was and that he would go a long way in the musical world. At first Simon could not believe it, in fact none of us could quite comprehend it, but it did make all the family happy! And it made Simon stop arguing with Mum and Dad when they told him to do his music practise. Of course he took to the viola too like a duck to water. Although John Curro was my brother's music teacher for just two years he became a great family friend. And that connection still remains to this day with John, now in his mid 80s.

Chapter Eleven
Around Our Swimming Pool!

My physiotherapist was talking to Mum one day and asked if we had ever thought of putting in a swimming pool. "Hydrotherapy would be so good for building up Marg's muscles. If you do this she will be walking by herself in no time," she said.

Mum and Dad discussed the possibility that night around the dinner table. He liked the idea, in fact that weekend Dad and Eric looked for a suitable site. Because our back yard was so huge, it took a while to find the best location. Hard working as they were, they knew when they had been beaten, this job was too big for them. The next week Dad rang some sub-contractors and it took ages to build the in-ground pool. Once installed, it was left to Dad and Eric to tile the top and sides, which they could only do on weekends.

To me the pool was so much more than a way to make my muscles stronger. I will always be grateful to my parents for building it. Our pool was a way to improve my communication skills and social life as well as the strength in my legs and arms. On afternoons when there were only a few others in the pool I would do laps and a lot of walking practice. The repeated body movement greatly improved my fitness and stamina, and probably kept me mobile for longer. To this day I love swimming and go whenever I can.

Swimming pools are people magnets. Every afternoon after school, teenagers from our street and nearby would come over for a swim. This is what they told their parents they were doing but really there was more jumping and splashing going on.

In those days it was pretty rare for families to have a swimming pool in their backyard. Many an afternoon it had its work cut out for it and I was in the thick of it, dog paddling right into a huge rinse of water from seven or eight friends (male friends of course), dive bombing each other. It was like a watery warzone with me in the middle joining in all the fun and egging them on. I know that my physiotherapist did not have this in mind. Still it was an awful lot of fun being a 12-year-old girl hanging out with a group of teenage guys.

We did not always jump and carry on like complete idiots. Sometimes we were quite sensible in the pool and used it the way it was intended. It all depended who was with us. Simon used to swim for Brisbane Grammar School, so he would train in his own backyard. Chris and Dad both enjoyed a dip in the pool because they too liked keeping fit. Even Mum got in occasionally.

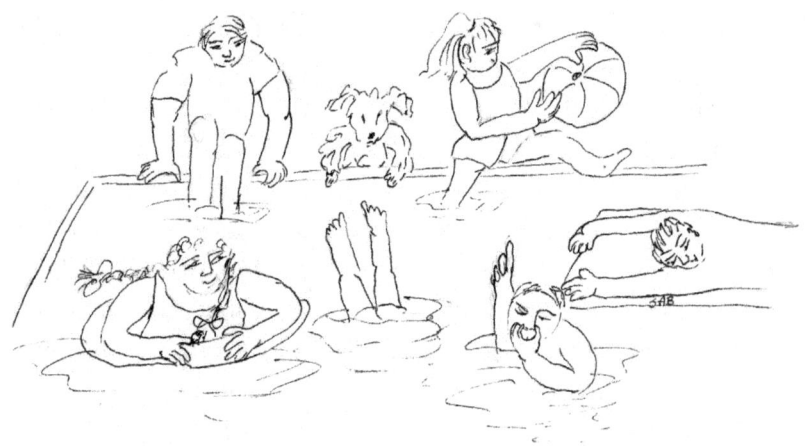

Mum had made a friend called Mrs Giles, who lived down the road with three daughters, aged from 11 to 18 years. Mum thought it would be good for me to have some girl company of my own age. As usual she was right. The next weekend was very hot so all three of them decided to venture down to our place for a swim. I was so excited to have new friends. Over time they gained my confidence until I joined in their discussions but they could not understand me at first. During the next few weeks, I kept trying to talk to them, and they were trying to work out what I was saying. Then one Saturday, we were sitting on the edge of the pool drying off, talking about school and it all fell into place. It was the very first time that anyone outside our immediate circle had been able to understand me. Boy, it felt great to be able to communicate with other people.

It took us about six months to get over the death of Pam. Then we started asking Mum and Dad if we could have another dog. After a lot of discussion on what kind of dog we should get this time, we all decided to take our chances with a Labrador retriever, that we called Jasper. There was no doubt our dog was quite intelligent, but he had a wilful way about him. If we told him off for eating one of our shoes or doing something horrible, he would straight away turn around, and go downstairs to worry a certain patch of garden which was always torn to pieces.

These dogs love to fetch things and so there were times when I would be in the swimming tyre in the middle of the pool.

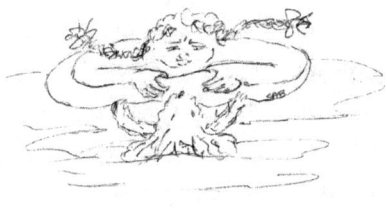

Jasper would start barking loudly as if to say "Get over to the side". I totally refused to be told what to do by a dog! After barking a few minutes he would jump in the pool, push me over to the side and hop back out again. Frustrating!

Moving to New Farm meant other new life opportunities for both Mum and me. I was occasionally invited by the hostel matron to accompany them on picnics and other excursions. One of these outings was to see over a battle ship, which was quite an adventure. At the beginning of 1970, matron asked if I would like to go horse riding every Saturday morning. I jumped at the chance of escaping from the house and trying something new. As it turned out I was quite good at riding.

Living only five minutes' drive away from school also meant I could have physiotherapy before class, at half past eight in the morning, instead of having it during school time or, worse, during religious studies. This really suited because instead of having treatment by myself, which was quite boring, I had it with two of my best girlfriends.

Mum had not resumed her teaching career since having children, until one day Mr Swan asked if she would mind doing some supply teaching for him. After thinking it over she gave it a go and enjoyed it so much she decided to become the relief teacher at Newstead Opportunity School, where I used to go to learn how to sew and cook – although because of my hand function this was mainly a social activity for me. After two or three years of juggling teaching with looking after everyone, she became a full time teacher when I was in my late teens.

My teenage years were some of the happiest days of my life but they were also some of the darkest. I can remember Mum telling me "Remember the good times, and forget the bad times".

Those were the days of the 'rat-pack'. We called ourselves that simply because we were like rats – we enjoyed good food, the best wine, living it up. We refused to talk about mundane stuff like how we could earn a crust. We would not talk about school. This privileged group was made up of Mum, Dad, Simon and Chris and I, and a couple of close friends. Almost every Friday night we would go out somewhere for a meal, but mostly we would go to a fish restaurant in the valley.

These nights were always a joy. I well remember my eighteenth birthday party at a German restaurant in downtown Brisbane. It was quite an intimate party, about 15 of us, and Simon knew the piano player at the restaurant, so he and his girlfriend Karen took along their violas to add flavour to the occasion. When we first arrived, we were well-mannered and polite, like any other group looking for a good meal and a good time.

But as the eating and drinking went on our behaviour went to the pack. It was very late when we left the restaurant and by this time we were all very drunk, to say the least! Even with two people to help me, on the way out to the street I still fell head-first into a rubbish bin!

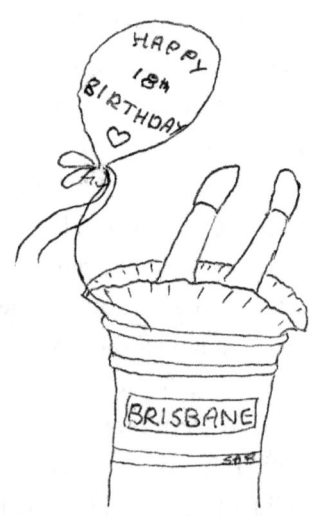

Chapter Twelve

Starting To Follow Our Dreams

Early in the 1970s, my physiotherapist told me I would be going into a new treatment group, but not just any old group. This one was based on a new technique from Hungary, called Conductive Education.

It was the brainstorm of Andras Peto, a fellow who was interested in anything and everything that affects mankind. This direction of his life probably came from having a father in a wheelchair, due to Parkinson's disease. During the Second World War, he returned to Budapest where he spent most of his time working and playing with his young daughter, who just happened to have cerebral palsy.

After the war ended in 1945, Peto started working on a carefully integrated system of coordinated exercises to better balance every part of our bodies. These exercises were based on observations of his daughter's condition. Conductive Education is based on the belief that the nervous system has the capacity to repair itself. For me and my Thursday morning physio group the session was only an hour a week, it was far less intense than in Hungary. Using this system of treatment, I made good progress and really enjoyed it.

When Brisbane hosted the National Physiotherapy Conference in the early 70s, I was asked to help demonstrate this new method of treatment at New Farm Spastic Centre. I can well remember this proud day, being a part of the practical demonstrations. At first a team of four of us did the mat exercises on the floor, and then we climbed up on chairs for the sitting exercises. What we showed them greatly interested the delegates, and I guess some of them took these techniques back home to use with their clients.

Now my classmates and I were close to leaving high school. To prepare me for this time, I spent a year in the Spastic Centre workshop for two hours a week. This was where we would pack items for different companies, such as ice cream spoons and lawnmower parts, while some other clients used to make seagrass mats.

I naturally thought that I would be going over to the workshop full time when I finished school at the end of that year. That was until my occupational therapist had a talk to me. She explained that my hand function was still very slow and she could see that I had to really concentrate to get the job done. If I decided to go full time after the Christmas holidays, she felt I would find it extremely tiring having to focus so hard all day, five days a week. When she told me this, I thought deeply for a minute, and then looked at her blankly because I really wasn't sure what to do.

She suggested I spend a year in a special vocational training unit directly opposite my school, and gave me a week to think it over. I talked to my parents, as well as my friends, and decided to go into the special training unit, as I thought it might give me a lot more variety and the opportunity to meet new people.

Our routine in this unit included three days a week of contract packing work at our desks, for about two hours at a time. We were always invited to join in with any activities around the school because most of the people in my class were from that school anyway.

However, the best thing by far was that I did not have to go to physiotherapy three times a week. Instead I only went to physio once every three weeks, or when I needed to go. Looking back on it, this was not a great idea. Only a year later, the muscles around my hip started to tighten up and I was still putting my hip out when I walked.

During that year, I started to study with the Secondary Correspondence School. This I was really excited about. The first subject I took with this school was 'Business Principles'. I don't know why I decided to take a subject to do with maths because I have never been any good with numbers! All my friends gave me a hand with the maths component of the subject, so it was not too bad and I passed without any problems.

This was also the year I managed to

throw away my boots, which were unfashionable things. When my physiotherapist told me I didn't need to wear them any more I let out such a scream of delight. That Saturday morning Mum and Dad took me shopping and I bought two pairs of sandals and two pairs of shoes - including a red pair. It was so exciting! All in all it was a really great year, a year when I had the best of both worlds.

Although my future was pretty well in hand at the time, Simon was having his own problems. He knew what he wanted to do, but it wasn't as simple as that! One day after we had spent the morning working in the garden, I was taking myself up the back stairs when there was a roar from Dad, "Simon, did I hear what I thought you said!" Simon and Dad were yelling about something. Then I heard Simon shout back more, about moving down to Hobart at the beginning of next year to study for a degree in music. There was a look of complete horror on poor Dad's face. If I could have run and hidden under my bed, I would have!

With fire burning in his face, Dad thundered, "I did not bring you up for 16 years to throw your life away going into a career where you will never know if you are going to make it or not. I always planned for you to go to University of Queensland and do architecture like I did after the war, so that you can take over my architectural practice when I am too old to work."

This outburst from Dad brought Mum running, "Frank, you know as well as I do that Simon is very talented. As much as you would like him to follow in your footsteps, he has too much talent to ignore." Mum often came to our rescue when Dad got going and with this very firm word he soon calmed down. Then he could see the sense in my brother's argument, and why he wanted to go down to Hobart, where the best strings teacher in the country was based. Ever since that day, Dad (or Frank as my brothers now called him) was very supportive of Simon wanting to be a musician.

As always, poor Chris was the one who did not know what he wanted to do. High school is difficult for many students. But for my second brother, every subject was a struggle, except for English, his favourite subject, which he passed quite well. For his entire school life, Chris' worst subject was maths, and the poor kid really didn't like this subject. When he was in Grade 7 at New Farm State School he was so frightened when he went into a maths exam that he ripped the exam paper. In high school, he was privately tutored in maths and German, so he could get a reasonable pass in his senior year. Doing more study after that final day at school was not in his nature, but he had no idea what he wanted to do with his life, except he was interested in boats.

For a while he did a few odd jobs for Mum and Dad. Then Dad got him a job as a builder's labourer on a pub site. Dad was the architect for this job and it was in Redcliff.

This didn't worry Chris. Right from the time he was a little boy, when he decided to work he worked hard, whether it was making a model aeroplane or sailing. He would get up at 5.30am and make his breakfast, then drive to work to the other side of town until the construction job was finished.

An old friend of ours, another Neal, had a barge for driving piles into the river and Chris was keen to work for him. To begin with they were working on the jetty across from our own, so until they moved on to another job all he had to do was get out of bed, eat breakfast and walk down the backyard. Chris really enjoyed working with Neal for a little over two years, until he could not employ him anymore. So he took a job with a very good friend who had a big laundry in Hamilton, and fitted his sailing in around it, as well as nights out with the boys.

In 1977, Queensland had a really right-wing Premier, Joh Bjelke-Pedersen. He was also a member of the Liberal Coalition, and was a real character. During the 70s, the political climate in Queensland was like a bomb ready to go off. There was a tour of the Springbok rugby football team from South Africa at the time when apartheid was a big issue, and Joh declared a state of emergency because the general public was protesting against the issue. There were a lot of power cuts at the time, to try to stop people from protesting, and it was a tense time for everybody. As a result, Chris had to work all sorts of hours, to get people's laundry done when the power was on.

Chapter Thirteen

New Directions For The Future

By now Dad had been an architect for more than 30 years. He loved his job and had met so many people in that time that he really enjoyed working with. But it was time for him to branch out just a little from architecture. He went into property development on Bribie Island, in Moreton Bay. This small island is about an hour's drive north of Brisbane, and is 34 kilometres long and eight kilometres wide.

Before 1963, everything the island needed, including its people, came in by barge. I think this boat was called the *Koopa*. Then the bridge across Pumicestone Passage was built, opening up the island, and it became a thriving community and popular retirement and holiday spot.

Dad had met a retired sea captain on the Brisbane bayside, who was a builder by trade. They decided to form a partnership in developing a huge amount of seaside land, and made a great team for a couple of years. While Dad had the knowledge to design and clear the blocks, Jim had the knowledge to build houses and home units on them. While this partnership lasted the two families shared a few dinners together down at Royal Queensland Yacht Squadron and one day we went for a really memorable picnic right in the centre of Bribie Island.

One morning we woke to the sad news that Jim had killed himself with an old shot-gun during the night. Of course his wife Mary and her two boys were devastated when it happened.

After Jim's funeral, she had to find a way to support herself and her two teenage children.

Until this happened to Jim, it never dawned on me to even think about what Mary did before she married Jim. I got such a surprise when the workshop physio asked, "Do you and your family know a Mary who lives near the Royal Queensland Yacht Club?"

I replied "Yes, but why?" The physio said Mary was a physiotherapist, and had applied to work at the league in the adult area. "This means the she will be working with you. How do you feel about working with Mary?"

Of course it did not worry me because I had found her to be a nice person on the several times we had met. So she became a member of our Thursday physio group.

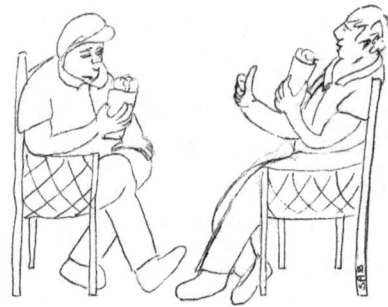

After Jim's death, Dad had to find another partner to continue this land division. He searched everywhere for about a year, then heard of a retired sugar cane farmer from North Queensland who had just moved into New Farm. When Dad went to see him, he quickly agreed to join up.

When he introduced his new partner Marcus we straight away fell in love with him and nicknamed him 'The Little Man' because he was about five foot tall, just skin and bone but he had an aura about him. He was about Dad's age, or he could have been a bit older and was one of those blokes who could turn his hand to anything.

He had decided to move his family to Brisbane to give his two sons more career opportunities – one went on to study dentistry and the other wanted to be a financial planner.

As I said before, Mum went back to full-time teaching as a domestic science teacher for two years until, once more, she got high blood pressure problems again. Now at her age it was quite serious and harder to control. I was fast becoming concerned about this as she had always been there when I needed her, and when my brothers needed her too for that matter.

As a mother she was very protective of me, especially when we had to go out together and see someone about my welfare. A very good example of this was when I went to see a medical specialist of any kind, she would talk on my behalf by explaining to the doctors what the problem was. Towards the end of her life this made me very frustrated with her because I knew she was not getting any better and one day she would not be there to take me to these appointments, and that really frightened me. The mere thought of this made me feel very nervous indeed because the writing was on the wall now. Some nights I would sit in my room after going to bed and ask myself *What will life be without her??*

Chapter Fourteen

A Crisis Hits The Family

In January of 1972, Simon moved down to Hobart to study for his first music degree with Jan Sedivka, one of the country's foremost violin teachers, at the University of Tasmania. He was from Prague but gained special merit for his contribution to contemporary music in Australia. We were all very sad to see Simon move so far away from home, but we all knew that he had a real talent that just had to be developed.

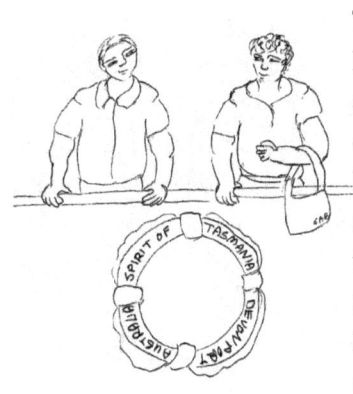

Towards the end of the year, seeing Simon had done so well living away from home and passing his music exams, Mum decided to fly down to Hobart, have a holiday and see the sights of Australia's smallest capital. After a delightful week, they set off for Devonport to catch the ferry *The Spirit of Tasmania* back across Bass Strait to Melbourne. Yes, Simon was coming home for the holidays!

After 11 hours on the ferry, and two days on the road, in what they described as a "dream run", they rang up mid-afternoon to say they were in Warwick and we would see them around 7.30pm.

Half an hour from home it started to rain quite heavily. Simon, who was driving, had no way of avoiding another vehicle when its driver lost control on a corner and hit them head on. Simon walked away from the crash with an injured knee. It was very lucky for all of us that the accident occurred close to Princess Alexandra Hospital, one of the largest hospitals in Brisbane, because Mum had multiple severe injuries.

By 8pm we were starting to wonder where they were. When the phone rang, Dad jumped up to answer it as if he knew something had happened. It was then he was told there had been a crash and Mum was in a bad way. Not only had the seat belt caused serious internal injuries but her car seat had been crushed on impact. Her spleen was bleeding badly, one of her lungs had collapsed and kept filling up with fluid, which was very dangerous. She also had a broken collarbone, seven broken ribs and her back was injured in many places. Poor Mum was just clinging to life.

Five minutes, later Dad rang a friend to come and look after Chris and I, so he could go to the hospital. When he arrived there he found out Simon was okay, except for a broken kneebone. On the other hand, poor Mum's injuries were so grave she had to have emergency surgery later that night to repair her spleen and collapsed lung.

I heard the garage door open later that night as Dad came home. By this time I had been fed and put to bed but sleep just would not come. I was too distressed. I heard Dad talking to Chris, then he and Simon they came into my bedroom. After I gave Simon a big hug they told me that Mum was in a very serious condition, and I burst into tears. They assured me everything would be all right so very soon I settled down and went to sleep.

I did not wake up until quite late, by which time Dad had already talked to the hospital to find out how Mum was. The report was serious but stable. The four of us had quite a lazy morning because we were all very tired after a very late night. Sometime during the morning Dad asked me if I would like to go and see Mum. The mere thought of seeing her in intensive care made me feel very scared indeed. So I said I would rather wait until she came down to the ward.

Simon had to rest his knee for a week. When Dad and Chris left for the hospital we decided to go in the pool. Swimming around, I started thinking about the last 24 hours in my life and trying to make sense of it. The friend who was looking after us had overcome many problems in her own life, so I started talking to her about Mum's injuries and how I was feeling. Out of the many thousands of cars which travel on that busy Brisbane main road, why did a drunk driver hit Simon and poor old Mum's little car? I think I was panicking and many questions were going through my head. Questions like *what would happen if Mum didn't get better and couldn't look after me? What if she got worse?*

When they came home late afternoon, Dad seemed more distressed than ever because Mum's condition hadn't changed. Soon after, he headed for the beer fridge, got himself a stubby and went down to sit on his boat. Another of Dad's character traits was to take himself off somewhere, where he could sit and think by himself. Besides being very worried about Mum, I was becoming worried about him because he seemed to be bottling everything up instead of talking about it. But this time our friend didn't allow him to be alone. She too went to the fridge and got a wine for herself, a coke for me, and we joined him on the boat.

Life is very strange! Although all three of us had been through a huge emotional upheaval in the last 24 hours, there was such a beautiful sunset over the river it gave us a real sense of peace, so that we could think clearly. Up to this point in my life I think that this would be the worst thing that had happened to me. Mum was my best friend and principal carer, especially when my father wasn't around. I looked over at Dad and wondered what these 24 hours meant to him. Mum and Dad had been married more than 30 years, for him I think it was the possibility of losing a wonderful wife and partner. When she was able to come home, he didn't know how much she could do, or when she would be able to do it.

After being in intensive care four days, Mum was well enough to go down to a ward. I was pleasantly surprised to see her looking so well when Dad took me up to see her. She was complaining about her broken collarbone and her back. She didn't mention her ruptured spleen and damaged lung, which must also have been extremely painful.

The next time Dad took us up to the hospital was on Christmas morning. The four of us took her presents and she was in one of her jubilant moods. There was wrapping paper everywhere, and we tucked into the hospital's really beautiful lunch for patients and their families. Once we had eaten them out of food and sung a few Christmas carols, we headed home after a great day.

Five days after Christmas, Mum was allowed to come home. We all thought she would make a full recovery in time but, sadly, she never did. In time her broken collarbone repaired itself, but she was still in an enormous amount of pain. When the back passenger seat hit the front seat it damaged all the disks in her spine and, because of her age, she very quickly developed spinal arthritis.

Before the accident Mum was a fairly active woman. During 1971 and 1972 she worked as a supply teacher both at my school and Newstead Opportunity School. As well as these two jobs she would sometimes play croquet with one of her elderly friends on Wednesday mornings. This sport is a bit like snooker, but played on an open lawn.

Although Mum grumbled about having to take her friend to croquet, I think she enjoyed playing and getting out in the sunshine. We all knew straight away that she would never be able to play croquet again because of her injuries.

Chapter Fifteen

The Next Few Years

When school went back the next year, Mum decided that she was well enough to go back to supply teaching. Dad and Chris agreed to do more of the jobs around the house because we knew that she had to rest her back as much as possible. I also agreed to help as much as my disability allowed me to do so. This was no trouble because we all really enjoyed helping Mum, after all she had looked after us all our lives.

For a few years Mum's health was fairly good considering the number of injuries she had sustained. However, soon afterwards her blood pressure started to go up once more and we all knew only too well that this could lead to her having heart problems. Mum being Mum was not prepared to give up just yet. In 1976 there was a domestic science teacher position at New Farm Senior School. This was her speciality so she decided to take it.

Consequently, the next couple of years were pretty busy for the whole family. In their free time, Dad and Chris went sailing on Saturday afternoons and sometimes overnight. They used to race to every part of Moreton Bay and then have a great party overnight and race back the next day. I did not mind them sailing just in the bay off Manly because I knew that they would be safe. But when I knew they were sailing offshore, I felt very worried and edgy.

There was one thing we did not like, and could not get used to in the years Mum lived after the car accident - Dad's cooking! From 1978, Mum would only cook three nights a week and Dad would cook dinner the other days. Mum was such a good cook, she could create almost anything. Dad was just the opposite, the only things he could cook were chops, eggs and steak. And only ever two vegetables - potato and pumpkin.

My first year working full-time in the workshop was a very busy one as I was also continuing my secondary education, studying English through the correspondence school. Mum helped me with this, being a teacher herself. However, there was also a very tiny education unit as part of the workshop. This was run by Mavis Scott, the wife of Bill Scott, an Australian folklorist, songwriter and folk history collector. She had a keen interest in the written word and every Thursday afternoon she ran a group for anyone interested in exploring their creativity. It was Mavis' support, as well as encouragement from family and two other writer friends, that nurtured my interest in writing.

I spent as much time as I could out of the workshop and in the education unit. This was because the contract packing work and envelope-stuffing for businesses around town was downright boring. I was quite excited when I started working in the handcraft section on Tuesdays and Thursdays because this was a lot more enjoyable. We made big colourful baskets woven out of plastic, and also used to tile the tops of tables. I found my fellow employees more interesting there, they were more talkative about more absorbing topics, like what was going on in the world around us.

There was lots to talk about. Those were the days when Premier Joh Bjelke-Petersen was on a control mission to keep people in their place. When Australia was pulling out of Vietnam, and Gough Whitlam became the country's first Labor leader in 23 years. There were public scandals like the firebombing of the *Whisky Au Go Go* nightclub in Brisbane, that killed 15 people, and an opinion poll that made 'Advance Australia Fair' our national anthem – even though none of us could remember the words! And on the tennis court, Evonne Goolagong sensationally won the Women's Singles at Wimbledon against another Aussie Margaret Court.

The dream of not having much physiotherapy in my adult life was very soon put to an end. A few weeks after I started full-time in the workshop, the physio mentioned her concerns about the way I moved my left hip. At that time I was still walking totally by myself but I sensed this was important, so we talked for more than an hour.

She explained that now I was 18 and no longer a child, the way I placed more weight over my left hip was going to cause it to tighten up as I got older, and this could become very painful in years to come. All this came as a bit of a shock but I wanted to know what could be done about the situation. She suggested I come to see her three days a week to try to improve the way I was walking. This treatment was very painful and at night it would be sore. As it turned out, I don't think the treatment helped my hip much, or the way I walked.

Not long after, the head of the workshop called me into her office to ask if I wanted to do some typing for a woman who regularly did interviews with her employees but could not type quickly herself. I was really enjoying working in handcraft but this was too good an opportunity to miss, so I decided to type for Pat three days a week. I had learned to type when I was about five years old, of course, to help me with my schoolwork, so it's a skill I have had almost all my life, and a very useful one.

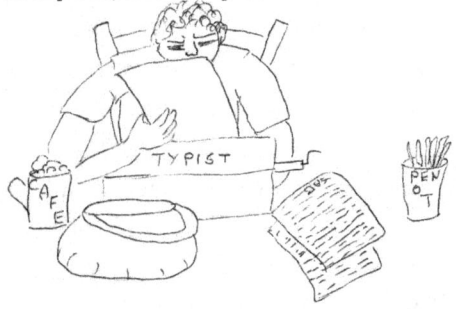

I earned a living both from my typing and the workshop, and looked forward to my pay packet every fortnight. What did I do with the money? Like any other teenage girl I bought music and clothes. Bell-bottom trousers and knickerbockers were my favourites.

In September 1976, Simon married a fellow violin player Karen Grimmer, whom he had known for 10 years. During his marriage to Karen they had a small hobby farm close to Hobart, in the beautiful Huon Valley. They even had a horse and led a self-sufficient lifestyle, growing their own vegetables.

In my first two years in the workshop Mum decided to give up work full time because she knew her health could fail in the next few years.

By that time I felt I should establish some goals for my life. My parents were getting older and it was important for me to know how to keep myself as comfortable as possible. To my mind, there would be three objectives. Firstly, I would have to work on my mobility to maintain a healthy body and mind. The most important thing to me was physiotherapy. This was something I would need for most of my life because of the way I walked, which is the case for many people with cerebral palsy.

Secondly, I wanted to study many subjects with the Secondary Correspondence School so that I absorbed as much knowledge as I could because I wanted to do something special in life.

My third goal was to enjoy myself as much as possible. I guess this was a reaction to Mum and Dad always seeming to be pushing me to try new things, but to do them their way.

Throughout my life I have always found that I work better when I do things in my own time, at my own pace. For example, in 1977 Mum wanted me to do the whole of Grade 8 English with the Secondary Correspondence School in one year. It was indeed a lot of work but I completed it because I knew they wanted me to. However I had to work on this course most of the weekend, just about every weekend.

I was lucky to have brilliant parents but they did some things which, in hindsight, I cannot for the life of me understand. Maybe they felt they had to keep me fully occupied and challenged, or maybe underneath they were just very proud people and simply didn't see that I would take longer to complete a goal than Chris or Simon.

Chapter Sixteen
Life Goes On

Conditions for the disabled have changed enormously in my lifetime. Until the 1980s, most people with any kind of disability were looked after by their immediate family and friends. Once their family carers died they often had no choice but to go into an institution.

Without our long-suffering parents, most of us would have been stuck in bed all day, without being able to feed or clean ourselves, let alone be a part of the mainstream community.

I grew up in the era of the 'Medical Model,' which mostly focused on people who were ill or infirm – and that is how they thought of us. Whenever I think of this scheme, my blood runs cold. Instead of concentrating on the strengths and capabilities of the real person behind the disability, the people in charge believed we could be cured, or at least improved. The reality is we just have to make the most of what we've got – there are still no cures and, in many cases, few improvements.

Then came a decade of change, starting with the United Nations declaring 1981 to be the International Year of Disabled Persons. It called for governments and the community to change the way they treated the disabled. The slogan for the year was *"A wheelchair in every home"* to highlight the rights of people with disabilities to be included in everyday life.

This was the start of a quiet revolution that is still taking place. I was 24 at the time and had been working for years. A young woman, definitely too old to be treated like a baby. It used to make me feel embarrassed, and a bit appalled, at the way people reacted when confronted with disability...and it still does.

Hundreds of events were held around the country that year, and brought disabled people together on an unprecedented scale. Previously they had mainly kept to their own groups, so this opportunity gave them a more direct way to be seen and heard, and to get their message across. All we wanted was a bit of dignity and respect, and a lot more practical support.

When I heard about a large rally planned in Brisbane, so big it was being held at a major boys' school, I asked Dad to drive me there to see what I could do, not quite knowing what to expect.

There were four big 'lacks' being discussed that day – not enough suitable supported accommodation in the community, no meaningful work so disabled people could earn a normal wage instead of living on a pension, better education and improved transport.

Transport was the one I was interested in. Maybe I knew one day I would have to rely on taxis to take me places. Speaking up was a real test for my speech but that did not worry me in the least, and it gave me a good idea of how effectively I could communicate in public.

While the first of the disability reforms that would make my life more comfortable in years to come were gradually starting to take shape, there was a fair bit happening on the home front.

At the beginning of 1979, Simon had been on tour overseas. When he came home to Hobart he discovered his wife had left him. Mum and Dad suggested he come home to Brisbane for a while until he recovered from the shock. For the first two months he didn't do anything much except seeing his old friends. Then he started to think about what he wanted to do next with his life. So, after talking to his friends, he decided to go over to the United States to study for another degree so he could teach music. The two-year course he chose was a Master of Arts in Music at the University of California in San Diego.

Meanwhile Chris had been in the workforce for some years and had no intention of returning to study. His whole life continued to revolve around his work and sailing, but when he lost his job at the laundry sometime around March 1985 he also decided to go over to America, to the west coast, to try and get a job as a deckhand. For once in his life he had good luck, because he landed a job as captain of a 50ft yacht, and was known as 'Captain Chris' for quite a few years.

In June of 1985, it was very certain that poor Mum was not going to recover from her high blood pressure. This could no longer be controlled by medication alone, so red wine was also prescribed to try to keep it in check.

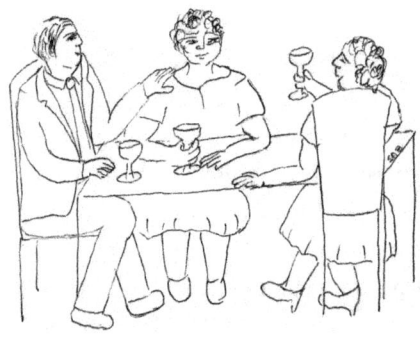

In September, Dad started thinking ahead about what to do for Christmas, and had one of his better ideas. By this time Mum was too unwell to prepare Christmas dinner with all the trimmings. Seeing it could be the very last Christmas Day we would have together, he decided we should go to the excellent Park Royal Hotel to celebrate with a slap-up lunch. I am so thankful we did because I have so many great memories of that day. We were all relaxed and happy, the food was really delicious and we had Christmas carols to entertain us.

That was not all Dad did in September. He went to see Mum's doctor to find out if she was well enough to go away to Melbourne and Hobart for three weeks. Surprisingly he was told that she was not too weak to travel down to see her sister Irene in Melbourne, then journey on to Tasmania to see Simon and his new bride Victoria. They had moved back from the States so he could take up an appointment teaching music at the University of Tasmania.

I was thrilled when Dad told me we were going down south mid-January, because our extended Christmas break would give me a whole seven weeks' holiday from work.

As I think back to our week in Melbourne, it is a time I will always treasure; the three of us were away from Brisbane, away from the pressures of life – spending precious time with Mum. I can remember Dad pushing my wheelchair around Toorak and along Chapel Street, my eyes wide open as we walked past all the exclusive boutiques and trendy shops. Another day we went to Melbourne's botanic gardens with Irene, and had a wonderful time wandering through the grounds. It was just so relaxing, four people enjoying one another's company and the best that nature can offer.

For some unknown reason, all three of us felt a real sense of sadness as the plane began to travel down the runway. It was like Dad and I felt the pain in Mum leaving her sister, perhaps for the very last time.

In no time we were off the ground and flying towards Tasmania, a bit apprehensive about how we would communicate with Simon's American wife. Although we all spoke English, we seemed to be worlds' apart. And they were probably wondering how they were going to cope with us!

They welcomed us at Hobart Airport (which is minute compared with Melbourne and Brisbane airports) and took us home to their very tiny house at Battery Point, right in the middle of the city.

On this trip we really did not do too much travelling. During the day we worked around the house and then went out to dinner at night. One day trip we did take was to Ross, in the middle of the island, halfway between Hobart and Launceston. Like many Tasmanian towns it is loaded with convict history.

One night Simon and Victoria took us out to dinner with some good friends of theirs, who just happened to live in a round house they had designed and built. Nowadays these houses come in kit form in whatever colour you want but back then they were pretty unusual. I had never seen or heard of a round house so I was as interested in the building as the company. These friends were also from San Diego, belonged to the same church as our newlyweds and were fun people. We were all quite disappointed to have to go home so early that evening, but were worried about Mum overdoing things, as she had not been well that day.

Next day we went out to a nursery nearby to buy some plants that liked the morning sun. They decided on azaleas, then asked Dad's advice on what sort of Balinese-style gazebos to buy for the garden, as their former strings teacher wanted them to host a party at home to welcome new students to the university's music department. Once that was all sorted, we went up Mount Nelson for lunch. We had been there many times before but not for a meal, and had promised Mum we would eat there, as she loved the outlook up there so much. The café was called Mount Nelson Signal Station, just 10 minutes from Hobart, with sweeping views over the Derwent River. We spent a couple of hours having a long lazy lunch and a walk in the station grounds, determined to make the most of our togetherness.

Chapter Seventeen

Out Of The Blue

A week or so after we returned home, Dad and I walked into the house to find Mum sitting in a chair on the back veranda. She told Dad to put on the kettle as she had some wonderful news to tell us. When the coffee arrived, she told us she had seen her physican Dr Joe Stroll that morning to see how the holiday had affected her blood pressure. To their complete amazement, it had gone back to normal after all this time.

"Mum, that is wonderful news," I cried. "I also have something to tell you and Dad." I explained that I had been talking to my physiotherapist Robyn about our adventures. When I asked her about the ongoing soreness in my hip, she suggested examining me in her rooms the next day, and then referring me to an orthopaedic surgeon to find out where the pain was coming from. Mum and Dad agreed it was high time to do something about the problem because it had gone on long enough.

As well as seeing the physio next day, I also saw my speech therapist Joan. Surprisingly, she was quite pleased with the progress in my speech while we were on holidays. The good news was I would only have one appointment a week with her this year. This was a great result because Joan was a pretty controlling woman at times, but I knew her well enough to see she was really a kind, gentle person and that I was part of her family. There were times when she took me home to her place for outings or overnight, so I came to regard her as a friend. But there was a catch. The bargain we clients made with her, in exchange for less speech classes, was that we would start rehearsing a play of her choice (knowing Joan this concerned me quite a bit). However we all knew a deal was a deal and we just had to go through with it.

As it turned out we needn't have worried. The play she chose was "*Peter Pan*" and I got to be Tinkerbell, which was great fun.

My mother rang the physio to tell her she totally agreed that I should see a bone specialist about my left hip. Now that she knew she would be around a lot longer, she wanted to see me free of pain. She went on to tell Robyn that I had not seen an orthopaedic surgeon for years, not since I was about 10 years old.

I have my first memory of an X-ray when I was about that age. I was so afraid because there were so many strange machines in a very small room. Believe you me I was happy when they finished taking images of my hips that time and Dad could lift me off that really uncomfortable bed and carry me out of that room.

With that decision made, something inside me felt a lot easier knowing that Mum and Dad would both be there for my hip consultation. If I needed an operation, Mum could support me through it, now that she was well enough. Not that I wanted a hip operation if I didn't really need one and, as it turned out, it wasn't necessary.

The rest of the week Mum was very happy, in fact I think during that week she was the happiest she had been in a couple of years. She was certainly busy, maybe too busy, planning for the future.

Monday morning came around, with no indication that there was anything amiss in our little household that would change my life forever. Dad was off to Bribie Island for a couple of hours, but would be back for a late lunch. I was off to work, like I did every Monday. I don't remember what I was doing on that day, it was an ordinary day until I was on the bus on the way home. Just as we approached the block of flats on the corner opposite our place, I got a terrible pain in my tummy, as though there was something terribly wrong at home. As the bus pulled up at my place, just as it had done so many times before, I saw a big black old car outside. *Hold on,* I said to myself, *that's Dr Stroll's car, what on earth is it doing here?*

Then I saw the doctor and Dad coming out to help me off the bus. As Dad opened the door, the doctor stroked my hair as he said, "I am very sorry Marg, but your mother died at 1.30 this afternoon, as she was having her lunch."

I didn't know what to do. It was as if I was fixed to the spot. They helped me into the house, and into my room, and the doctor stayed with me while Dad got a drink of milk to calm me down.

Then Dr Stroll told me about a conversation he had with Mum. She knew that she was awfully sick and her blood pressure could go up and down at any time. She knew the unexpectedly normal pressure reading might only last a short time. Her main fear was to have a bad stroke and end up in hospital for a long time.

My mother Glenda Mavis Oswell died of a heart attack on 24 February 1986. She was a wonderful woman, a completely devoted mother to my brothers and I. She was my friend, my rock and my protector.

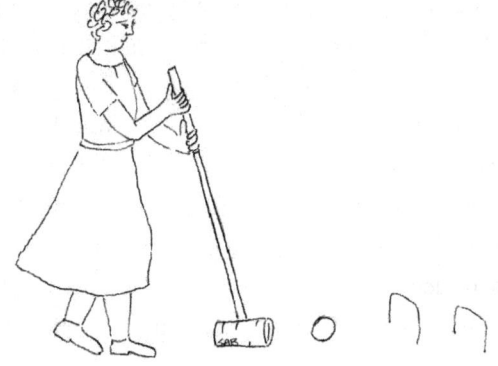

Chapter Eighteen

One Foot In Front Of The Other

They say when one door shuts, another door opens – and it opens wide.

Since Mum's death I have known my fair share of fear, and my share of wonderful events, being family and otherwise. I was heartbroken when she died, but life didn't stop. Fortunately, there has always been someone to support me and help state my case, especially after the death of my father.

Dad lived for another 17 years after Mum's death. He wanted to keep me at home but, after a few weeks, it was too much for him. Together we made the hard decision that I would move out to Sunnybank, on the other side of the city, to live in a share house with three other disabled people.

Looking back I can see now that this change was the making of me. It allowed me to become independent and resourceful while still having family to look out for me, to some extent.

For the first year or so, I was concerned about Dad. He kept telling me how little he liked living by himself. Then he told me that he had met up with a very old client, and asked if I wanted to meet her.

Like a two-year old jumping for joy I said "Yes please!" So it was arranged that we would go out to Bribie Island for the day to get to know one another. She wasn't really what I expected. But Margaret was a really gorgeous woman and I quite liked her.

A few months later, Dad was taking me back to Sunnybank after I had spent the weekend with him and, without much emotion, he said, "That was your last weekend at home, because this week Margaret and I are going to sell the old house. I have already bought a small unit in East Brisbane, near her place. She is the best thing that has happened to me since your Mum died."

"Do Simon and Chris know about this?" I inquired. This time he took a few minutes to reply, as if he was thinking about the best answer to give.

"Marg, there comes a time in everyone's life when you have to please yourself, and stop doing whatever people want you to do. So we have decided not to tell Simon or Chris until we have sold the house and I have moved into my unit."

It was my turn to think long and hard. Then I said, "Yes, now that you have pointed it out, I agree. You deserve to be happy, Dad".

This was the best day in years, or so I thought at the time. Later I needed to put on a brave face because I had very mixed feelings about what was going on. It was the start of a very challenging period in my life, finding my own way. I am grateful to have grown up in a well-to-do family, but I now know money is not everything. You just need enough to be comfortable, so you can get on with life the way I have.

When I first moved away from home, my flatmates and I had a house mother to coordinate daily arrangements and do the grocery shopping. This wasn't a bad system, much better than the awful alternative of existing in an institution, but it all depended on the personality of the individual in charge.

Later, when my friends and I were feeling more settled and self-reliant in our lives, we moved into a brand new group house. This time we chose to be helped by support workers, which gave us a lot more freedom.

About the same time there was a change to the way disabled people were employed. Instead of everybody getting paid the same for whatever we did in the workshop, and all of us having a weekly program of some contract work, some educational outings, some therapy, people were separated according to their hand function. It became illegal for those who were good with their hands to work in the same building with those needing more support.

The more able ones went to an employment service and worked all day. Unfortunately cerebral palsy sufferers with less hand function, such as myself, were forced onto different programs where we didn't get paid.

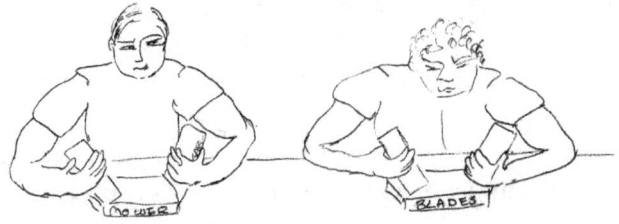

At the time I was working at the Rocklea Activity Therapy Centre, and living nearby. I didn't want to work full time because I knew I was a bit slow, but the alternative turned out to be quite boring and it did nothing for our self-respect.

Thankfully my hand function still gets me by for my day-to-day needs. I can easily pick up a book to read, set myself up to use the computer or do some study, as well as doing other simple little things.

In 1995 I became actively involved in a lobby group to get better transport services from the government. This group was called '*Transport and the Disabled: how to achieve more choices and options for getting around the community*'. It started up after the Australian Disabled Standards was written, and was part of Queensland's United Nations reform process.

This group had plenty of momentum, thanks to an amazing woman called Roslyn. She wasn't disabled, she just wanted to help and was passionate about our cause. Ros acted as our secretary, did all the writing and recording, and held the group together with her gentle good humour and commonsense.

She made sure everyone had the same chance to be heard. At first she would make me repeat myself until the others understood what I was saying – and sometimes it took a while for them to cotton on. We took things very slowly but were determined to communicate well. Everyone in the group was of the same mind about the things that needed to be done.

At the time I had a boyfriend named Ian. He too was disabled, after an accident left him with limited movement down one side. I got to know him through the transport group, and we gradually became friends. There was something about him, I was a bit wary at first. He was a bit impolite about women but he was funny and he made me laugh. We were really close for a year, and went out and about together, but ultimately he and I wanted different things out of life. Nevertheless, we stayed friends until he died of cancer some years later. He was an interesting man and I'm glad I had the chance to know him.

I continued to be involved in the lobby group for a while but eventually stopped going because I find these sorts of meetings physically taxing and very often it takes a long time to get things done.

Our transport group just sort of petered out over time. Some of the most active members, including the wonderful Roslyn, died. But I think it achieved what we set out to do, over time governments heard what the disabled community was saying and have provided more services and support.

After many years of having the freedom to walk, my mobility changed dramatically. My whole body tightened up until I could not move a muscle. A lifetime of throwing my left hip out with every step I took had put too much pressure on my spine.

I was 41 when the main nerve in my back collapsed without anyone suspecting it. Ironically, two weeks before it happened, my doctor had ordered an MRI scan. They got to me just in time. Without an immediate spinal operation I would have been paralysed for the rest of my life. At least I got most of my body movement back, after three months in hospital having physiotherapy every day, although I now needed a wheelchair to get around.

Every disabled person in the community receives some sort of support package, but it doesn't cover the extra services they need to make them more comfortable and help them keep up their skills and capability. Physiotherapy is a good example. The pain in my hips and neck has got worse over the years, so I still have physio every two to three weeks. This special care doesn't come cheaply. If my father had not been able to make sure I had enough money, I could never afford regular treatment on a pension.

Sunday 21 October 2001 is a day I will always remember. It was the day the Goodwill Bridge opened, the first walking and cycling link over the Brisbane River. After joining the crowds to be first over the bridge with Dad and Margaret, we went back to their unit for lunch. About a week later he had a bad fall at home. Margaret couldn't get him up so she called an ambulance, which took him to the Mater Hospital just over the road from their place. Although the doctors couldn't find anything medically wrong with my father, he never recovered the use of his legs. He went into a nursing home, where he died on 11 August 2003 at the age of 83.

Meanwhile Chris and Simon have got on with their lives. Simon married for a third time, to musician Bronwyn Myers in January 1993. They were married in the City Botanical Gardens, right in the middle of Brisbane. Sebastian James was their first born in 1995 in Brisbane. At the beginning of 1996 they moved to Los Angeles for 10 years, where Simon was involved in the Hollywood music scene. Juliet was born there in 1997, and Ben came along in 2002.

In 2005 they moved back to Toowoomba after Bronwyn's mother Mary was diagnosed with colon cancer. I was living in a share house in Toowoomba at the time Simon and family were there, and it was a real help to have them close by.

These days, Simon and family live in Melbourne, his base for an active solo and chamber music career. Bronwyn is Head of Strings at Wesley College in Glen Waverley, while he regularly travels overseas to play viola for film scores, music festivals and guest artist performances. His career includes playing on the sound tracks of more than 800 films, from the Academy Award winning scores of *Schindler's List* and *Titanic*, to *Star Trek* movies, *The March of the Penguins* and, more recently, *The Railway Man,* for which Simon performed a number of solos.

Chris has remained in the United States, skippering yachts – except for a year back in Brisbane to help Dad with the Bribie Island land development. Then he returned to Fort Lauderdale, Florida and sailing life. During the global market collapse the yachting scene went very quiet, so he worked at Washington Dulles Airport as a scanning officer with Transport Security Administration. Now he is back at Fort Lauderdale again, working at the airport and planning to return to his beloved boats.

As for me, about seven years ago I moved to Victoria Point and have since found a wonderful place, close to the waterfront, to call my own. Since landing there I have created my own support network. I have many good friend and neighbours, a team of carers, and am blessed with the love and support of close family.

Since then I have discovered writing has no physical boundaries. It takes me anywhere I want to go and makes me anyone I want to be. This was my life-defining moment.

I am Marg Oswell – writer, thinker, student, fun-lover, wonky adventurer. Life is good.

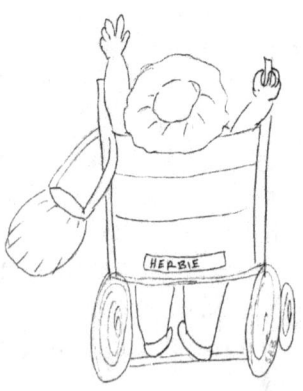

Afterword

A New Deal For Disabled People

There is no doubt the way disabled people are treated by the community and supported by the powers-that-be has come a long way. Like everything governments do, it is by robbing Peter to pay Paul. Yes, we are better off in a lot of ways. But (and this is a big 'but') it all depends on what services a person needs and what level of support disabled people are given. A support package includes the number of hours a handicapped person is attended by a support worker and this assessment depends on a medical report, written by a doctor employed by the same department that makes the rules and manages the funding.

We certainly have more basic recognition, thanks to a United Nations' Convention on the Rights of Persons with Disabilities adopted late in 2006, after four years of intense negotiation. It still remains the fastest international human rights treaty yet declared. When Australia accepted this convention on 17 July 2008, it agreed to protect people with disabilities from discrimination, ensuring equal treatment under the law and securing our human rights and fundamental freedoms. Looking back, the shift from a welfare system of caring for the disabled to considering their civil, social, political and economic rights has been a real turning point for community attitudes.

The lobby group I was involved in has changed over the years but still exists, to ensure the Federal Government kept its agreement to make all public places in Australia entirely wheelchair accessible by the end of 2015. This includes ramps at the entrances to buildings, level pathways in parks and gardens and wheelchair-friendly toilets. I am very proud to have been part of this movement to help disabled people be more mobile in the community.

As a disabled cerebral palsy person, I truly feel that the United Nations and other important policymakers have gone too far towards complete integration into the mainstream community. I think there should be a happy medium. Sometimes I think there should still be a choice if parents want to send their child to a separate school. I grew up going to what some people demeaningly called "special" school. We were a community, where we got our education, all our physiotherapy, occupational and speech therapy. These 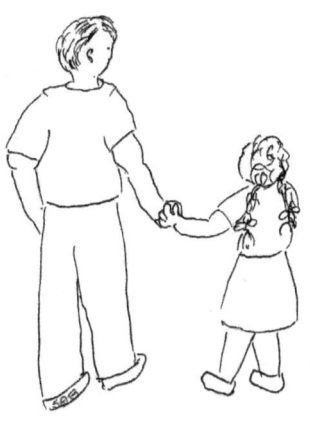 services were delivered as part of the weekly school routine, without our parents having to pay. In a sense it was almost an industry. But were we children segregated, I wonder? In my view, by the time you added all the therapists, the office staff and others who supported us, we were a community within the larger community of the suburb of New Farm.

Now, in 2015, we have another new deal for the disabled to look forward to and, in a sense, it's a bit like here we go again. The new national disability insurance scheme, Disability Care Australia, is continuing to be rolled out. Queenslanders won't see much benefit for a couple of years yet but the intention, finally, is to tailor individual support plans for every disabled person that are based around their potential as well as their long term needs.

I look forward to that day, and to a support system that is equal and fair for all.

Acknowledgements

To my family for always being there. My brothers Chris Oswell in the US, and Simon Oswell and family in Melbourne

Thank you to Chris Volker, my senior support worker at Toowoomba who got me started writing this book.

My carers Kylie, Julia, Shelly and Cheryl for helping me through each day, and Tracey my physiotherapist for continuing to give me as much mobility as possible.

The Cerebral Palsy League Queensland (CPL) and Connect2 for the resources they provide to enable me to be part of the community.

Special mention to Dorothy Uncles. She has been a physiotherapist for CPL for 25 years, and is always there when my wheelchair needs attention.

Thank you especially to Ruth Connor, Helen Irving, Michael Blaney, Frank Oschmann, Kaylene Tyrrell, Denis Neilsen, Lynda Smith, Bruce Kirkpatrick, all my other friends at CPL Capalaba Support in Community Centre, and the lovely Linda Sturgess who takes us out on Sundays.

To all my supporters, including Anna Cahill for her writing advice, editing and proof reading support, Susan Ballantyne of Dunedin, New Zealand for her wonderful, whimsical sketches

I am indebted to freelance editor Sonia Cahill for her long-distance advice and critical review of the text from Shanghai, China, and especially to the amazing people at Book Whispers who have brought my manuscript into published form.

To Tracey Walmsley, and all the therapists, carers, teachers, support workers and social workers, too many to name, that I have had the good fortune to know over the years – this memoir is my tribute to you all.

The Author

Margaret Frances Oswell grew up in Brisbane, Queensland. She and her trusty wheelchair Herbie now live at Victoria Point in adjoining Redland City. This memoir is her first book, some years in the making. Since she found her voice, she has studied creative writing and is off and away writing whatever takes her fancy.

The Editor

Anna Cahill is a professional journalist, trained in New Zealand, who now works as a editor/proof reader, communications adviser and writing tutor on Brisbane's bayside. She joined CPL's Capalaba Support in Community centre as a volunteer to help Marg complete her life story. Page by page, the content came together over two years, working in the shade of a huge mulberry tree (their 'tree of knowledge') in the centre garden.

The Illustrator

Susan Ballantyne is a self-taught artist, living and working in Dunedin, New Zealand. Art is her leisure pastime and passion. She regularly exhibits her work, which ranges from detailed botanical subjects to people and places, in a number of mediums. Commissioned to draw a series of sketches to capture moments in Marg's story, this is Susan's first venture into published book illustration.

www.ingramcontent.com/pod-product-compliance
Lightning Source LLC
Chambersburg PA
CBHW050543300426
44113CB00012B/2239